ANXIETY

Dominate Your Depression, Phobias, Panic and
Beat Social Anxiety With the Power of Cbt

(Overcome Social Anxiety and Negative Thought
Patterns Using Mindfulness Meditation and Nlp)

Robert Carbonell

Published by Kevin Dennis

© **Robert Carbonell**

All Rights Reserved

Anxiety Therapy: Dominate Your Depression, Phobias, Panic and Beat Social Anxiety With the Power of Cbt (Overcome Social Anxiety and Negative Thought Patterns Using Mindfulness Meditation and Nlp)

ISBN 978-1-989920-44-2

Legal & Disclaimer

The information contained in this book is not designed to replace or take the place of any form of medicine or professional medical advice. The information in this book has been provided for educational and entertainment purposes only.

The information contained in this book has been compiled from sources deemed reliable, and it is accurate to the best of the Author's knowledge; however, the Author cannot guarantee its accuracy and validity and cannot be held liable for any errors or omissions. Changes are periodically made to this book. You must consult your doctor or get professional medical advice before using any of the suggested remedies, techniques, or information in this book.

Upon using the information contained in this book, you agree to hold harmless the Author from and against any damages, costs, and expenses, including any legal fees potentially resulting from the application of any of the information provided by this guide. This disclaimer applies to any damages or injury caused by the use and application, whether directly or indirectly, of any advice or information presented, whether for breach of contract, tort, negligence, personal injury, criminal intent, or under any other cause of action.

You agree to accept all risks of using the information presented inside this book. You need to consult a professional medical practitioner in order to ensure you are both able and healthy enough to participate in this program.

Table of Contents

Introduction

Most people find themselves feeling anxious once in a while. However, anxiety can become a real issue once it starts interfering with your daily activities. Anxiety is one of the major symptoms of all anxiety disorders some of which are discussed below. But the good news is that anxiety can be treated easily using natural procedures, treatments and medication.

What exactly is anxiety?

It is natural for you to feel fearful or tense whenever you are anxious. You can equally have one or two unpleasant physical symptoms. For instance, you may find yourself dealing with issues like palpitations, fast heart rate, tremors, sweating, chest pain, headaches, dry mouth, fast breathing.

Part of the physical symptoms are caused by the brain which sends lots of messages down the nerves to different parts of the body whenever you are anxious. The nerve messages tend to make the lungs, heart and other body parts work very fast. Additionally, your body releases stress hormones like adrenaline into your bloodstream whenever you are anxious. These can equally act on muscles, heart and other parts of the body to cause some symptoms.

Anxiety is seen as normal during stressful situations, and can even be very helpful. For instance, most people will become anxious whenever they are threatened by a very aggressive person, or before a crucial race. The surge of nerve impulses and adrenaline which we often experience in response to very stressful situations can encourage a flight or fight response.

Anxiety is quite abnormal if you notice any of the following:

•   Is out of proportion to the stressful situation; or

•   Persists even after the stressful situation is no longer there, or the stress is minor; or

- Appears for no real reason when there is no stressful situation.

Chapter 1: Self-Rating Anxiety Scale

You can deal with the problem only if you can understand it. In this chapter you will find Zung Self-Rating Anxiety Scale. We will be using this test due to its proven accuracy and ease of use. This test was developed by Williem W. K. Zung M.D. to quantify level of anxiety person is experiencing.

The Self-Rating Anxiety Scale measures anxiety level using 20 questions based on 4 groups of anxiety manifestations: cognitive, autonomic, motor and central nervous system symptoms. Please indicate how much each statement applies to you based on the previous two weeks.

Each answer is scaled from 1 to 4. Please read questions carefully as some of them are negatively worded as to prevent set response. To sum up your score use the scale, which you can find below the test.

Take a piece of paper and answer these questions selecting which applies to you best: A; B; C or D.

A - A little of the time

B - Some of the time

C - Good part of the time

D - Most of the time

1. I feel more nervous and anxious than usual.

2. I feel afraid for no reason at all.

3. I get upset easily or feel panicky.

4. I feel like I am falling apart and going to pieces.

5. I feel that everything is all right and nothing bad will happen.

6. My arms and legs shake and tremble.

7. I am bothered by headaches, neck and back pain.

8. I feel weak and get tired easily.

9. I feel calm and can sit still easily.

10. I can feel my heart beating fast.

11. I am bothered by dizzy spells.

12. I have fainting spells or feel like it.

13. I can breathe in and out easily.

14. I get numbness and tingling in my fingers and toes.

15. I am bothered by stomach aches or indigestion.

16. I have to empty my bladder often.

17. My hands are usually dry and warm.

18. My face gets hot and blushes.

19. I fall asleep easily and get a good night's rest.

20. I have nightmares.

You have your answers so it is time to tally your score. Please calculate your score using this answer key:

1. A - 1; B - 2; C - 3; D - 4

2. A - 1; B - 2; C - 3; D - 4

3. A - 1; B - 2; C - 3; D - 4

4. A - 1; B - 2; C - 3; D - 4

5. A - 4; B - 3; C - 2; D - 1

6. A - 1; B - 2; C - 3; D - 4

7. A - 1; B - 2; C - 3; D - 4

8. A - 1; B - 2; C - 3; D - 4

9. A - 4; B - 3; C - 2; D - 1

10. A - 1; B - 2; C - 3; D - 4

11. A - 1; B - 2; C - 3; D - 4

12. A - 1; B - 2; C - 3; D - 4

13. A - 4; B - 3; C - 2; D - 1

14. A - 1; B - 2; C - 3; D - 4

15. A - 1; B - 2; C - 3; D - 4

16. A - 1; B - 2; C - 3; D - 4

17. A - 4; B - 3; C - 2; D - 1

18. A - 1; B - 2; C - 3; D - 4

19. A - 4; B - 3; C - 2; D - 1

20. A - 1; B - 2; C - 3; D - 4

Calculate your score to find out your anxiety level:

20-44 Normal Range

45-59 Mild to Moderate Anxiety Levels

60-74 Marked to Severe Anxiety Levels

75-80 Extreme Anxiety Levels

Normal Range

If you scored up to 44 points that means that you experience low levels of anxiety. You may have felt inclined to read this book because you felt a sudden spike of anxiety. If this was caused by a specific event like, for example, an upcoming public speaking event, you can learn tactics that will help you deal with these specific issues. Breathing and muscle relaxation exercises will help you relieve stress.

Mild to Moderate Anxiety Level

If you scored in a range of 45 - 59 that means that you experience elevated levels of anxiety in your daily life. Some changes in your daily routine and your diet are required. Follow advice and exercises which are provided in this book to lower your anxiety level to a normal range.

Market to Severe Anxiety Level

If you scored in a range of 60 - 74 that means that your anxiety level is high. Dealing with anxiety has to be high priority for you. Follow this program with dedication and persistence and soon you will notice your anxiety level drop.

Extreme Anxiety Level

If you scored above 75 that means that you are suffering from extremely high levels of anxiety. This level of anxiety is accompanied by a severe form of anxiety - panic attack. In the next chapter you will learn breathing and muscle relaxation techniques that will help you stop panic attack in it's tracks and eliminate them from your life. With the help of exercises, diet and lifestyle changes you will be able to reduce your anxiety to a normal level.

IMPORTANT

If your symptoms are mostly physical make sure to complete a physical exam in order to rule out physical issues.

Do you experience these symptoms:

- Severe lack of energy or drive.

- Flat affect (complete lack of emotion) along with slowed thinking and behaviors.

- Severe appetite changes, headaches, and sleep problems.

If you feel these symptoms you may be experiencing depression and you need to consult your doctor. Please call and arrange a consultation with your doctor.

! If you experience suicidal thoughts please contact your doctor right away !

Chapter 2: So What Causes Anxiety?

When we are stressed or have anxiety, our bodies release cortisol which is the stress hormone associated with our Fight or Flight response. Long ago, when we were still living in caves, anxiety is what informed us to dangerous situations that we needed to avoid in order to survive.

Without anxiety, people would have been more likely to have been eaten by a predator, fall off a cliff, get bitten by a venomous snake, or experience a similar fate. Anxiety then is something in our evolution that had the original purpose of helping us to survive our world. Fast forward to today and we find that anxiety is still with us even though all of the dangers that existed before our modern civilization are no longer with us like they used to be.

When we have anxiety, our bodies still release cortisol as our biological response to a perceived potential threat when it encounters a stressful situation or belief. This can be the case even if that situation or belief can't actually do us any physical harm. We may feel anxiety when we have a deadline due, or when we worry that we're forgetting something important, when we're caught in traffic and we have somewhere we need to be, when we're concerned about being able to pay our bills, or when someone we associate with stress approaches us In each of these situations, the body may treat what's happening as a threat, even if we aren't in any actual physical danger.

It goes without saying that nature hasn't quite yet received the message that times have changed with the advancement of society. Yet the biological response we feel to perceived future threats can still show up in our lives and wreak havoc with them.

The cortisol released when we feel anxiety not only affects our emotional state but it can result in a myriad of health symptoms including weight gain, making learning and memorization more difficult, increasing cholesterol and blood pressure levels, as well as negatively affecting our immune systems, and even our bone density.

It can even contribute to someone becoming depressed and just basically siphon off our feelings of vitality. With that being said, in our day-to-day lives there are different situations which might cause you to feel anxiety. If any of these situations makes you feel anxiety, take a note of it as your anxiety is triggered either by this particular situation (or a similar situation) or by the things associated with that situation.

For instance, if your boss causes you to feel anxiety you may feel anxiety whenever he or she calls your name because you associate your boss with a perceived future threat whether that threat actually ends up being real or not.. If tests cause you anxiety and you associate studying with tests, and your anxiety is severe enough, it's possible that even the idea of studying might make you anxious.

When it comes to Social Anxiety, or the anxiety that you may feel when you encounter people, one of the reasons that you may have this kind of anxiety is that most people feel the need to be socially accepted by other people. As a result of this need for acceptance, we may fear others' disapproval and we may feel anxiety as our biological response over the idea that we may or may not get approval.

This is one of the main causes of Social Anxiety which in its extreme forms can interfere with a person's ability to form meaningful relationships or connections with other people. On a neurological level, the parts of the brain called the amygdala and the hippocampus get activated when we feel anxiety.

The amygdala is the part of the brain that regulates our emotions like anxiety and fear and the hippocampus is the part which has to do with forming memories related to emotions. When we feel anxiety, it is because we have learned to associate certain thoughts, beliefs, situations, or stimuli with being potentially threatening to us.

When we encounter similar thoughts, beliefs, situations, or stimuli, the amygdala and the hippocampus get activated and our body produces cortisol which makes us feel anxiety.

Chapter 3: Get A (Social) Life

So, you've decided you want to meet others and you know how to start going about it. And yet, you might find that you lack the confidence to find and keep friends so how do you cultivate that confidence?

Building Confidence

If we use the Oxford Dictionary again, the definition of 'confidence' is:

'(noun) – A feeling of self-assurance arising from an appreciation of one's own abilities or qualities'

As you can see from this definition, it can be totally feasible to be an introvert and to be confident. We have already established that shy people may well fear social interaction whereas introverts are more likely to feel exhausted by meaningless interaction.

The first step is to recognize which definition best describes you. Is your lack of confidence making you unhappy? Do you want to establish relationships with others? If so, then you need to do something about it and this might well involve you in stepping outside of your comfort zone and making that first move.

Of course, you might feel challenged by this so start off with small challenges like the ones we've already discussed: say hello, start a conversation with a co-worker.

As well as getting to know others, it's just as important to start getting to know yourself. What motivates you and gets you excited? What would get you out of bed on a cold, wet day? What do you believe in? What would you like to achieve? What would make you proud of yourself?

No-one should know you better than yourself and self-discovery can make for a fascinating journey. You could start keeping a journal to put yourself more in touch with you and make you more self-aware. You have to learn to love yourself before anyone else will appreciate you. Try meditation to find peace with your own thoughts and refuse to listen to negative self-talk. Watch out for any triggers that threaten to push you into them, recognize them for what they are, surplus to requirements, and move on.

Really listen to what others are saying and learn how to find common ground or even constructively challenge when possible to open up your vistas and theirs.

Confidence is not necessarily being outspoken and loud. It is not about being an extrovert. You are you and should accept yourself for who you are, warts and all.

In today's world, introversion is, wrongly, undervalued. Introverts can be misconceived as boring because they are quiet. They are sometimes not considered to have anything to 'bring to the table.' But that need not be the case. Do not be prepared to be submissive. Show people how much you have to offer and start with small steps. Watch the tone of your voice, your body language, and your facial expressions and try to ensure that you display an assertive impression. Walk tall; don't slouch as if you're trying to hide. Start by smiling when you're on the telephone; a lot of us loathe using the phone but a smile can actually be detected over the telephone. Start using it and notice the difference.

And then practice, practice, practice.

Building Social Skills

To start with, you might need to stretch your boundaries and this is when it comes back to capitalizing on your hobbies or obsessions. You have so much knowledge around these subjects and probably have a lot to say. You can share this with like-minded people.

Learn to observe the body language of others. Are they just being polite or have they turned to you, genuinely interested in what you have to say and are anxious to share what they know with you? If they are just being polite, simply move onto the next person.

Remember to be yourself, you are already very familiar with whom you are and this is a continuous work in progress. Be authentic. Everyone has something to offer. If the person you are engaging with seems bored, maybe it's them who is boring. Or maybe you just haven't found the right person to be talking to. Or maybe you're in the wrong place altogether. Chalk it up as experience and move on to the next place/person/conversation.

Make your conversations a two-way interaction. No-one likes having to talk all the time without any feedback; it becomes tiresome for both parties. Learn to recognize cues for you to respond or offer up your contribution to the conversation. Of course, you will not be knowledgeable about everything, all the time. That's what makes social interaction great: we are constantly learning about others, about ourselves and about the world around us. Learn how to take advantage of it.

By interacting with others, you may well find you are more fulfilled emotionally, physically and socially.

Chapter 4: Learning More About Social

Phobia

There are many factors that can cause social anxiety, and they are grouped into: psychological, biological and environmental.

1. Psychological. The disorder or recurrence of your anxiety may be due to a traumatic experience in the past. It can be a humiliating social incident, getting bullied, or being neglected by those whom you considered as friends.

2. Biological. You are more likely to develop the disorder if a first-degree relative has it or battled with it. This can also happen as a result of certain abnormalities in the brain circuits, specifically the parts that are responsible for controlling the emotions and handling a person's fight or flight response.

3.   Environmental. The fear may evolve from seeing how other people were embarrassed or humiliated in public. Children who were raised in a sheltered manner and were not taught proper social skills are prone to develop the disorder.

The Stages of Social Anxiety

1. Infancy to early part of adolescence

The condition is said to be a normal part of a person's developmental growth. It first occurs during infancy. This is actually an important stage to go through because it can hone a person's social skills as he/she gets older.

A person is bound to experience repeated social anxiety attacks during the latter part of his/her childhood until early adolescence. This is due to the cognitive development and more frequent exposure to stress and pressure.

Adolescents suffer from social anxiety mainly due to issues with peers, self-consciousness and public speaking. This can also happen as a result of a traumatic past experience that continues to haunt the person when he/she needs to be in the same position. In most cases, adolescents learn from all the experience and surpass the stage by meeting with the demands and social pressure.

The sad fact remains that the number of children diagnosed with the disorder gets higher through time. This can lead to bigger problems if the symptoms will be ignored due to lack of information. This can cause a person to lose interest with his/her studies or in going out and making friends. It is not easy to determine the symptoms, especially when you are monitoring a child's behavior. You have to get the help of a professional to determine if your child is just painfully shy or is already showing signs of social anxiety disorder.

2. Adults

It is easier to spot the condition in adults. Some of the most common behaviors include having stage fright, shying away from any social activities, and keeping to themselves most of the time. The need to get tested and medically cured is determined by the intensity of one's social anxiety. When it becomes too uncomfortable to the point that the behavior is already interfering with one's progress, then this is a clear sign that you ought to get a professional help.

How is the disorder diagnosed?

You must first consult with a general practitioner who will assess your health. He/she will ask questions about your medical history in order to make an evaluation. You will be asked to have a physical exam. The doctor needs to make sure that nothing else is bothering you aside from the anxiety.

There are no laboratory tests involved in the procedure, but your doctor may recommend other tests if he/she suspects that the condition may be a result of a physical illness. You never know, but the painful shyness may come as a result of how your body responds to an illness that you may still not be aware of.

The doctor can give you proper medications or recommend that you go to a mental health professional, like a psychiatrist or psychologist. These doctors are capable of asking the right questions in order to identify the roots of the problem. The evaluation period is not easy. At this point, you will be prompted to remember the details and memories of the past that are haunting you and are causing your anxiety.

You must never hold back. Your doctor is trying to dig deeper in order to understand where the problem is really coming from. You have to help your doctor in understanding the situation; what led you here, what has caused the condition, and what triggers the symptoms.

It may take a number of sessions before the doctor's verdict is finally given. This is to ensure that everything has been covered and the doctor understands the intensity of the disorder and the duration of the symptoms.

Chapter 5: How Anxiety, Stress And

Worry Effect Children

Naturally as we get older our levels of experience grow and we develop a sense of perspective. We also become more secure in ourselves and our decisions, often because as we go through the many up's and down's life throws at us we develop a feeling "everything will work itself out" – and it normally does.

Children don't naturally have the same outlook and as a result what feels like a fairly small issue to you may well be a massive one to your child. If they are showing the signs of stress or worry this is an important factor to consider.

As with most things in life, prevention is better than cure. By fostering a relationship of open communication with your children before anything is up you can gain great benefits in the long haul as your children will feel able to approach you.

There can be numerous reasons why we don't develop that kind of relationship and can even be something as simple as embarrassment on our part.

If we take sex as an example, most kids start sex education at aged around aged 12. We can simply leave it to their school to take care of and we don't need to get involved, however if we approach the subject as they are first experiencing it at school and let them know that you are not embarrassed to talkabout"how babies are made" the lines of communication are open. If at 13 or 14 your child is starting to have an interest in sex and possibly has a partner who is putting pressure on them to have sex they will be more likely to speak to you rather than keeping it pent up and getting stressed over it.

Some of the key indicators that your child may be stressed or anxious are as follows:

•   Change in appetite or eating habits.

- Loss of interest in school and schoolwork, possibly including worsening grades.

- Difficulty going to sleep or staying asleep (insomnia).

- Frequent stomachaches, headaches, or other excuses to stay home from school.

- Sudden withdrawal from family activities.

- Change from happy and secure to moody and depressed.

- Torn or blood-stained clothes.

- Damaged or lost property, particularly mobile phones.

- Change in the groups they usually hang out with, especially if friends suddenly stop coming around.

- Sudden need for extra money.

- Increased anxious or nervous behaviour.

• Spending more time on the computer or the phone and not wanting you to see what their doing online.

Gently approaching the subject may get your child to open up, that's often a better option initially than outright sitting them down and giving them the third degree. If you're too direct it's likely they may clam up however body language alone at the point you ask them the direct question maybe all you need to gain a decent idea if anything is up.

The need open up the lines of communication and starting to help resolve any issues is paramount, the following list is in no way designed to be scary or to make you worry but being aware of the potential seriousness of childhood stress is important.

Issues that can occur include:

• Depression

• Physical ailments (headaches, stomach aches, ulcers)

• Sleep problems

- Academic problems

- Frequent switching of schools

- Low self-esteem

- Weight loss or gain

- Long-term emotional scars

- Serious physical injury

- Property damage (possibly to their home or school)

- Problems with future relationships

- Violent aggression

Next we will begin to look at the most specific scenarios that cause anxiety, school avoidance and stress along with considering the key aspects of each and how we can prevent or solve the issue.

Chapter 6: Signs You Are Struggling With

Anger

Daily annoyances are driving you crazy

Do you get mad occasionally? Then it's totally fine, but if you find yourself losing it over every little thing that doesn't happen to your liking on a daily basis, you have got a big problem. For instance, when I was dealing with my own anger problems, if my roomie forgot to unload the dishwasher, I would yell at him or give him the silent treatment. If you have a habit of yelling over the phone or find yourself road raging when you fight with someone, it's a strong signal that your anger has become out of control.

Things can get pretty intense with you

You don't just get mad you get really MAD. Now this is what I mean by intense anger. This is also a great barometer for analyzing an anger problem. Be honest with yourself and answer this. How intense do you get when you are angry on a scale of one to ten, ten being extremely calm, with zero being intensely enraged. If you rate yourself anywhere beyond 5, it's time for some heavy damage control.

You tend to hold grudges

Do you still get angry at the slightest mention of an old friend who did you wrong? If a considerable amount of time has passed since the incident happened, and you still can't seem to let go it, you should know that it's extremely unhealthy. Emotions aren't supposed to last more than a few minutes, hours or days. If we are holding on to our angry emotions for much longer than this, it's often called a grudge – something that can eat your peace away.

You get abusive quickly

If you swear at the drop of a hat, or get violent even at the slightest of provocation, chances are that you are a short fuse who can't control his or her anger. If you get to the point of being physically or verbally abusive more than once in a year, it says a lot about your mental state - which is extremely problematic right now. Being out of control is not a feeling anyone enjoys, and you should look at your behavior as an opportunity to change yourself.

You push friends away

If you are always angry, chances are that your friends might hesitate to call you. But it's also possible that you are the one who ends up pushing your friends away because you are not sure how to deal with your frustration. Experts believe that it's quite common for people to isolate themselves while they are trying to manage their anger issues.

Your heart starts racing when you get upset

Do you feel sick to the stomach and feel like your heart is racing? Then there are other physical symptoms such as shortness of breath, profuse sweating or headaches. If you experience these symptoms on a regular basis, it's time to take a serious look at whether it's a medical condition you have or it is your unhealed anger that's sending such destructive signals.

You feel overwhelmed

Trapped anger can leave you feeling empty. So don't be surprised if you feel exhausted, or unhappy because it's your anger that is causing you to feel overwhelmed. Have you been depressed lately? Chances are that your depression is masking itself and comes out as anger. If that's the case, seek immediate medical help without wasting any more time.

You apologize a lot

While apologizing all the time can also be a sign that you haven't forgiven yourself for something you did, most often it stems from unhealed anger. If your loved ones have been pulling away from you lately, or you spend most of your time trying to make up to them, you anger issues could be getting worst. You may also feel like you spend a large amount of your time fixing your relationships rather than maintaining them.

You are always defensive

How do you react to honest conversations? Are you always on the defensive? It has been observed that people who struggle with anger issues can have a really hard time seeing the big picture, and that causes them to turn defensive even at the slightest of jabs taken at them. And God forbid if someone calls them out for your anger that could mean unleashing all their frustration upon the other person in the worst possible way. Defensiveness is a common way of hiding one's anger or painful emotions from the past.

Your memory is always fuzzy

Anger can affect a large part of how your brain functions. Watch out for cognitive issues. Intense anger can spike your cortisol levels that can quickly turn into memory issues and being unable to create new memories. If you have noticed that you might be suffering from memory issues of late, it's more than time to work on releasing your anger or see a therapist who can help you overcome it. I promise you that you will have a much better life once you get past your anger issues.

Chapter 7: What Happens Through Your

Day

What is your daily anxiety cycle?

What are your daily triggers that raise your anxiety levels and in some cases bring on a panic attack?

What time of day is your anxiety at its worst?

When are your panic attacks most likely to occur?

Most importantly when are you the strongest? When is your headspace in control? Early morning, middle of the day, evening, through the night?

Step outside yourself and take a look. I have drawn a graph that shows the highs and lows of my daily anxiety.

24 hours of my life

My 24 hours explained

6-9am – I feel strong and can really stay in the now and see anxiety for what it is. I do all my planning at this time. I get the family and me organized for the day and usually feel really good.

9am – School drop off. Slight rise in anxiety as I may have to talk to people or I may be late. What if people look at my kids and don't think I am doing a good job? Usually these thoughts are pretty simple to stop at this point.

9:30 -2pm – Exercise. Doing household stuff, working on eBooks or websites, catching up with friends. Mornings are usually fun and not filled with much anxiety and I rarely have a panic attack in the morning.

2-6pm – Anxiety starts to build through the afternoon. Blood sugar has a low in the afternoon and this makes it worse.

I think about:

What I need to cook for dinner.

How can I juggle the afternoon activities?

Have I got enough food for tomorrow lunches?

Anxiety is not internalized yet and is pretty much dependent on what I have to get done.

6-10pm – Anxiety starts to build the more tired I become. It is now very internalized.

What a rotten job I have done today.

Kids haven't done reading for days.

Kids haven't done homework for 2 days. They will fall behind and it will be my fault.

I am such a bad mother.

I'm such a failure at everything. Who will want to read what I write.

I'm so tired all the time.

I'm such a useless mum; I can't even keep a clean house.

The list could go on and on but you get the idea. I have started to really internalize everything. The voice in my head has turned from what I have to get done to who I am as a person, mum, partner and manager of this family. This is my constant battle. My fight.

10pm – Sleep time. I have got this routine down really well. I have practiced relaxing, distracting my mind and pretty much fall straight to sleep.

3am – Nightmare time. If I wake up or get woken up by the kids I am instantly in a panic state.

Heart rate is fast and pounding.

Breathing is fast and shallow.

Feels like someone is sitting on my chest.

Muscles twitching especially in my arms.

Head space in chaos.

This panic used to stick around for a couple of hours. I would finally get to sleep and have to get up again to get going for the day. Not a great way to live.

Your 24 hours

Keep a journal of each day for a week to get an idea of when your anxiety rises, falls and spikes are. It is important to write it down this information as this will help us set up the fight plan that will be specific to you. You may not need to keep a journal as you probably already know when your feelings of anxiety are nonexistent and when they are at their worst. This will become the basis of your graph.

To do this,

• List times down the side of a page.

• Beside each time, write the events you had to go to or the tasks you had to do.

• Beside each of these, list a number out of 10 to describe the level of anxiety you were feeling. You can also use some key words to describe what your body and mind were doing at this time.

Levels:

0 Feeling great. Anxiety level is not registering.

1 Anxiety is barely there. Still feeling good.

2 Slight increase in the nervous feeling but still easy to ignore.

3 Nervous feeling increasing.

4 Anxiety symptoms are constant now and are underlying everything but tasks can still be done and thoughts are still clear.

5 Starting to become a bit frazzled.

6 Anxiety showing in increased heart rate, increase in nervous feeling and in thoughts feeling slightly confused.

7 Anxiety is internalized about who I am and how useless I am. Basic tasks seem overwhelming and thoughts are jumping everywhere very confused.

8 Anxiety is totally distracting and distressing. Feel very overwhelmed with everything. Panic is starting to creep in on top of the anxiety.

9 Panic attack is starting to increase intensity.

10 Full blown panic attack. Very difficult to concentrate on anything but the panic.

For example:

Time Task Level Body and Mind response

6-8am   Writing books. Getting me ready for the day. 0 -1   Body   relaxed, mind focused and feeling great.

8 – 9am   Getting kids ready for school.   2   Heart rate increased, still focused but conscious of anxiety starting to increase.

9:30am   School drop off   3

Anxiety increasing but still very manageable. Can fight it easily.

The next step is to transfer this information into a graph.

How does yours look? Can you see your most anxious times and when your panic times are? Writing it down helps distance the anxiety from who you are. It gives you the power back.

Knowing when the different high and low points occur during the day also gives you the opportunity to be prepared.

When you are stronger you can set yourself up with a fight plan (Ch 4) to be ready for combating this anxiety and panic. This fight plan will give you confidence throughout the day and take away the anxiety about becoming anxious. Look for signs of spike and follow your fight plan. Stop it before it starts.

I am not my anxiety.

I am not my panic attacks.

I am a strong confident woman, mother and person.

I put anxiety and panic out of my life.

I welcome into my life, peace, calm and a feeling of being organized and in control.

Chapter 8: Boosting Self-Confidence

To become more self-confident is easily attainable, provided that you have the attention and willpower to carry on with these things. The things you'll do to enhance your self-confidence will also increase your success level – your confidence will come from real, concrete achievement, which nobody can take away from you.

Below are the three steps which helps to build self-confidence:

Preparation; Set the Goals; and moving towards achievement.

Step 1: Preparation

Firstly, you have to prepare yourself to build confidence in yourself. You are required to think about where you wish to go, get yourself in the right state of mind for building self confidence:

In preparing, you need to conduct the five things mentioned below:

Look back on what you've previously achieved:

Think about your past, and then make a list of ten best things you've achieved so far (Achievement list). Perhaps you played a main role in the central team, came top in an important assessment, or did something that made a tremendous difference in somebody's life.

Make a document, which can be referred to anytime. And then spare some time weekly enjoying the accomplishments you achieved!

Consider your strong points:

When you look at your Achievement list, give a thought of what your friends will considers as your strong points and weak points. From here, you can think about the fear and opportunities you would face. You need to be sure that you take pleasure in looking at your strong points.

Think about what's significant for you, and where you would like to go:

Next step is to think about those things that really matter to you, and the things you want to accomplish in your life.

You need to set and achieve goals and true confidence would reflect from this. Setting a goal is a process in which you use to set objectives for yourself, and assess your successful attempts by striking those objectives.

Start organizing Your Mindset:

In this stage, you should start organizing your mind. You need to learn to overcome the pessimistic self-talks which can hamper your confidence.

And lastly hand over yourself to victory:

The final and last part of preparation is to give a clear assurance to yourself that you are totally dedicated to this journey of self confidence, and you promise that you will do all that you can do to achieve it. Self-confidence is like maintaining stability. At one end, people show low self-confidence. At the other, people are over-confident.

If your confidence level is low, you'll keep yourself away from risks; and you may give up. If you're over-confident, you are ready to take high risk, and extend yourself ahead of your abilities. You may also discover that you are confident enough that you don't attempt seriously to actually do well.

One should get it right by having a balanced confidence based on reality and your actual abilities. With the correct and balanced self-confidence, you will stretch yourself outside your capabilities.

Step 2: Set the Goals

You can make a start from here, slowly, going towards the goal that you have set for yourself. By doing this you can boost the confidence within you.

Build the information you are required to succeed:

By setting up your goals, you can discover the skills you will need to accomplish them. And then see how well you can obtain these skills boldly. You just don't need to accept good-enough resolution – look for an answer, a class that fully helps you to achieve your goals and, preferably, provides a document or qualification which you can admire.

Concentrate on the fundamentals:

At the beginning, don't try to do anything complicated or don't try to reach for excellence – just take pleasure in doing simple things successfully.

Start with smaller goals, and grab them:

You can start with the small goals you noticed in step 1, cultivate a habit to get them settled, attaining them, and rejoicing that attainment. You should not make challenging goals at this stage; just acquire the habit of attaining them and rejoicing them. Slowly and steadily, start building up the achievements.

Organize your Mind:

Reside on the positive thinking, and keep rejoicing the success, and keep up the mental images well-built.

You should also learn to tackle failure and accept that errors that can occur when you try to do something novel. In fact, if you cultivate the habit of dealing with mistakes and take them as learning, you can (almost) begin to see it in a constructive light.

Step 3: Moving Towards Achievement

In this stage, you'll realize that your confidence level is increasing. You will see that you have accomplished some of the classes that you have started in step 2, and you should have abundance of victory to rejoice!

At this time you can extend yourself. Now, start building slight bigger goals. Raise the size and level of your dedication. And expand the skills into fresh, but related arenas. Be humble – don't get over-confident and don't exceed your limit. And you need to make sure that you don't begin to enjoy cunningness.

Provided that you continue extending yourself, but not excessively, you will discover your confidence level rising up.

Managing your self-confidence

If you are low in self-confidence, is it possible to do things that will help to change that? Is your self-confidence in your control?

While it may not seem so, if you are low in self-confidence, you can certainly do things to increase your self-confidence. It is not hereditary, and you do not have to be dependent on others to increase your self-confidence. And if you believe that you are not very proficient, not very smart, not very eye-catching, etc. ... that can be changed.

You can become someone who is worthy of respect, and someone who can pursue what he wants irrespective of what others say or do.

You can do this by taking control of your life, and taking control of your self-confidence. By taking actual actions that improve your aptitude, your self-image, you can increase that self-confidence, without anyone's help.

Below, are the things that will help you do all that. Here they are, in no particular order:

1. Prepare yourself.

This means grooming yourself. This would seem obvious to you, however, it's astonishing to see the difference it would make, if you shower and shave. It will enhance the sense of your self-confidence and self-image.

2. Dress well.

If you dress well, you will feel nice about yourself. You will have a feeling of being presentable, well doing and you will be able to deal effectively with the world. Dressing nicely would have a different meaning for every individual. It means, being casually dressed means to look nice and does not necessarily have to have an expensive price tag.

3. Edit your image.

We all have a psychological image created for ourselves in our mind and it reflects how much confidence we have in ourselves. This picture is changeable and is not fixed. You should change your own image by utilizing your mental photoshop skills. You need to figure out the way you perceive yourself and you can discover a way to change it, if it's not a good one.

4. Think optimistic.

You should learn the act of replacing the negative thoughts with the positive thoughts. Kill your pessimistic thoughts. Try a self-talk or fight the negative thoughts (mentally) and fill this place with positive thoughts and positive energy. For this, you need to identify yourself well. You should listen to your feelings and beliefs. You should initiate diary writing on yourself and around the feelings you have for yourself. Then analyze your thoughts about yourself. Just give a thought to good things you identified about yourself, these are the things which you are good at, and you like as well. Start visualizing your limitations (real or artificial limitations). Do an in-depth study of yourself and you will come out with better self confidence).

5. Act optimistically.

In place of just thinking optimistically, this needs to be taken into action. Action is vital to develop your self-confidence. Your actions should always reflects a positive path; take actions rather than telling yourself that you can't, be positive. Speak to everyone in positive manner, energize your actions. You will soon see the difference.

6. Get prepared.

Prepare yourself to beat the feeling that you will not be able to achieve something. Assume about appearing for an examination: if you have not studied well, you won't be confident in your capabilities perform well in the examination. However if you concentrated on your studies, you are prepared and you'll feel more confident. Similarly, assume life as an exam, and get yourself prepared.

7. Increase your competence.

By getting educated and practicing, you can boost up your competence level. For example, if you plan to become a skilled writer, you should start writing short stories, Journal, blog, or do some sort of freelance writing for someone. With every bit of document you write, you can better your writing skills. You may also dedicate some time from your daily schedule (say 30-45 minutes to start with). This would give you ample of time to practice and polish your skills and competence.

8. First set small goals and attain them.

Mostly people get disheartened as they were aiming for the moon from the beginning and were not able to achieve success due to no experience and confidence. Instead, aim for something that is more attainable. Set a target which you know can be accomplished, and then go for it and sense that feeling of happiness after attaining success. Now set another small goal and go for it. With every successfully achieved goal, you will feel better and superior in your skills and these achievements would make you feel relaxed and comfortable. This would also give you the confidence to set bigger and achievable goals.

9. Focus on resolutions.

You need to change your focus from a complainer, to non-complainer, to solutions instead of problems. It is one of the best things you can do for your confidence and your career.

10. Smile and be thankful.

You will feel instantly better when you smile, and it helps to be kinder to others as well. Be grateful to what you have in your life. Begin the day by thinking about some of the things you have to be thankful for.

11. Empower yourself with awareness.

Empowering yourself is one of the best approaches for building self-confidence. You can do that in a number of ways, but one of the surest ways to empower yourself is through knowledge. By becoming more knowledgeable, you will feel more confident and you can become more knowledgeable by investigating and studying.

12. Put your belief in their place.

It is believed that the average human has 65,000 thoughts every day, However, it is assumed that 85 to 90 percent of them are negative--things to worry about or panic. The point is to keep that negativity in proportion.

13. Get ready to rebound.

Know that it is not failure that hampers our confidence; it's not getting back up. Once we get back up, we've learned what doesn't work and we can give it another try.

14. Choose your buddy sensibly.

Your outlook be it negative or positive-- will be the average of the five people you spend the most time with, therefore, you have to be careful who you hang out with. Make sure you're hanging out with people who give confidence to you and lift you up.

15. Do your groundwork.

In nearly any situation, preparation can help improve your confidence. If you have to give a speech: Practice it several times, record it and listen. If you are meeting people for the first time, check them and their organizations out on the Internet, and check their social media profiles as well. "If you're organized and well equipped, you will be more confident.

16. Get relaxes and exercises.

Having a sound sleep, good food, and exercise affects both your frame of mind and effectiveness. Just simple exercise three times a week for about 20 minutes is good enough to make you feel relaxed and calm.

Chapter 9: Indications Of Low Or No Self-

Confidence

Very many people suffer from low self-esteem and lack of assertiveness. You are not alone. At the same time, very few people know that they are victims of this self-destructive psychological disease.

Not knowing that you have self-esteem issues is dangerous. You will accept your fate and take life as it is. The belief that you are worthless will prevent you from living your life to the fullest.

Some of the common indications of low self-esteem include:

1.   Always avoids eye contact while conversing with others

2.   Lacks the confidence to express opinions

3.   Moves out of a challenge and never has the courage to stand up to others

4. Always criticizes oneself - Nothing lowers your confidence more than being negative about your life. It is one thing for people to criticize you but when it comes to you, it is a totally depressing.

5. Unable to appreciate compliments

6. Being very humble

7. Feeling as if you have to always be superior

8. Evident arrogance, egoistic behavior and a high sense of pride

9. Poor body language such as looking downwards

10. Feeling low when in a group of people

The aforementioned signs of low self-confidence are not the only ones. If you tell people sorry after little mistakes, then you may be having low self-esteem. It is good to feel remorseful after you mess up somebody a bit but overdoing it may portray your inadequacies. In addition, if, after you have done a mistake you ponder over it the whole day, you need to enhance your self-esteem.

If by doing an evaluation you conclude that you have a shaky self-esteem, it is time to solve it before it becomes a problem. It is your life, thus it is your mandate to improve your self-worth. Sometimes, you do not need a professional to boost your confidence.

If you are a victim of depression out of low self-esteem, you need to seek specialist help. Do not wait until it is too late to handle your case. The best way to enhance self-esteem is by reversing the above symptoms. For instance, avoid feeding your mind negative thoughts and start thinking positively.

If you are one of those people who can hardly express their opinions, you need to get started on how to make your voice heard. With time, you will cultivate a high self-esteem.

Chapter 10: 16 Embarrassing Job

Interview

Mistakes That Will Make You Look

Unprofessional

Originally published on November 29, 2017 in Career Advice,

Career Etiquette, Interview Prep, On-demand Video Courses

In the fall of 2017, CNBC aired a show called The Job Interview. It exhibited real people interviewing for real jobs with real employers. There were 20 cameras capturing all the nerve-wracking nuances of an interview. And all the mistakes. Those of which you can learn from and not make in your own interviews.

However, if you don't have the trained eye of a career coach, you probably wouldn't pick up on many of the mistakes just by watching the show.

So, I took the first episode and broke it down for you to see the little things most job candidates don't know they're doing wrong. And to be fair, I'm also pointing out some of the things they did right.

If you want to see the 20-minute episode, it's now available on Amazon Prime (click here to watch).

The first episode is about a Florida-based accounting firm that's in the tech space called Xendoo. They were looking to hire a detail-oriented bookkeeper.

Below is my commentary at various time markers in the episode. See if you pick up on the same things I'm noticing. What can you learn from what you see?

What NOT to overlook (3:06)

One of the qualifications for the job is someone who is detail-oriented. You'll notice how the interviewers are pouring over the resumes, looking for the smallest of mistakes to determine if each candidate is indeed detail-oriented or not. One

64

interviewer noticed how on one resume the text was off just half a space.

My clients wonder why I nit-pick their resumes.

This is a perfect example of why I do. As I've said in my blog and in my video guides, employers are looking for reasons to throw out your resume. Not reasons to keep it.

What NOT to wear (4:27)

For the type of job this woman is interviewing, she should really be wearing a blazer over her sleeveless top.

Always dress professionally and in a way that is customary to the particular industry.

How NOT to shake hands (4:48)

While this next candidate is dressed appropriately, he did not give a good handshake.

Always give a firm handshake. Anything too limp or too strong leaves a bad impression, as the interviewer indicates.

What NOT to assume (4:58)

The candidate's response as to why he gave the female interviewer a gentle handshake compared to the firm one he gave to the male interviewer shows his lack of understanding of business etiquette. In business, gender is neutral.

The other thing this candidate did wrong when beginning the interview is he swiveled and rocked in his chair. You'll see this mistake a lot throughout the episode from many of the other candidates as well.

If you're ever offered a seat in a swivel chair in an interview, resist the urge to swivel!

What NOT to say (5:10)

This candidate starts off strong with her response to

"Tell us about yourself," but almost crosses the line with a little too much personal information.

You want to avoid discussing marital status, children, and other personal matters since it is illegal for the interviewer to ask you for this type of personal information. While her sharing of this info didn't seem to cause a problem in this case, it could very well be a turn-off for other interviewers because they may fear being accused of making hiring decisions based on the personal information the candidate provided.

What NOT to ask (5:35)

This candidate says she did her research (like all candidates should), but if you listen to the first thing she said she knew about the company, you'll see she made her answer all about herself. She talked about how convenient it is for her that the company is located close to her house. You'll soon see too just how poor of a job she actually did on researching the company!

Another faux pas committed by this candidate is she came out and asked a very personal question of the interviewers. Just like interviewers should avoid asking candidates personal questions, so should candidates avoid asking the interviewers personal questions!

What NOT to avoid (7:05)

This candidate did a good job of establishing rapport with the interviewers early in her interview.

Be yourself without getting too personal with the interviewer. If it becomes clear in the interview you have some of the same interests in common, feel free to use that as common ground to build rapport with the interviewer.

How NOT to answer "What do you feel is your greatest strength?" (7:22)

Do you know what each candidate did wrong in answering this question?

None of them gave an example of how they've previously demonstrated their strength. Always answer with specific examples, never in generalities. Providing examples makes you stand out in a positive way and makes you more memorable to the interviewers.

How NOT to answer "What would be your greatest weakness?" (7:30)

So what did all the candidates do wrong in their answers to this question?

They all listed a personality trait as their weakness instead of a skill. Why should you never answer this question with a personality trait? Because personality traits are more ingrained in us, and therefore take a long time to unlearn, if ever.

However, a skill is something that can be quickly learned or improved upon.

There are several other ways screw up your answer to this question, and several ways to answer it well.

Go to Chapter 5 to learn more about how to answer

"What's your greatest weakness?"

How NOT to behave (8:24)

We're now about to see how the candidate who said she'd done her research actually did NOT do a good job on her research.

She said she doesn't have the desire to go back into accounting, ALL WHILE INTERVIEWING FOR

AN ACCOUNTING POSITION! (REALLY?!!).

She didn't have a clue that the company or the position was related to accounting.

Plus her negative, flippant attitude about the industry and her inappropriate laughter about leaving a previous job were completely out of place and a turn-off to the interviewers.

What NOT to judge (13:20)

As shown here, interviewers aren't perfect and they too can make embarrassing mistakes in interviews.

Remember they're human just like you are, so don't let them intimidate you to the point that you can't perform and sell yourself to the best of your ability.

In fact, I notice how my clients become less nervous about an interview when I remind them that the interviewers are also nervous. Interviewers are typically nervous about making a wrong decision and therefore costing the company a lot of money, unintentionally letting an illegal or inappropriate question slip out, and making you feel more nervous than you probably are.

Approaching it this way can help you relax.

How NOT to fail the test (14:13)

Here you'll see the third or fourth test the interviewers have given the candidates. Always be prepared for potential tests.

For example, if you're going into sales, you'll probably have to sell something to the interviewer.

If you're going into a job that will require you to give presentations on a regular basis, you may be asked to prepare a presentation for your interview.

Years ago, I had a day-long interview where in one part of the afternoon I was given 45 minutes and certain parameters to come up with an idea for a new program that could be implemented throughout the organization. I then had to present on my idea and why it would be a good program for the organization.

I didn't get the job, and later found out that no one got the job. It made all of us candidates wonder if the company held interviews just to get ideas without having to pay a salary for them. This can and has happened before, which is a very unethical practice on the part of a company. If you ever sense this is what's going on in one of your interviews, consider it a red flag!

What NOT to include (14:39)

When given a test, never say, "I don't like being put on the spot," like this candidate did.

What NOT to leave out (17:04)

This candidate gave a good response to the question of "What would this job mean to you?"

So did the candidate at the 17:15 mark. I liked that she said, "I have a lot to give," instead of "I feel like I have a lot to give."

"I have" shows more confidence than "I feel like I have."

However, as the interviewer, I would want to know how has she given a lot and been an asset in her past experience? What are some examples of her giving her all and being an asset to her previous company?

I'd want to hear stories about times when she's demonstrated these qualities. Again, these stories are what make a candidate memorable.

What NOT to forget (18:18)

Here are the things the interviewers were most attracted to:

• Positive attitude

• Someone who "gets it"

• Someone who "wants it"

No matter how negative of an experience your last job was or your current job search is, leave all negativity at the door. Interviewers can sense a negative attitude very quickly so do what you can to improve your attitude before walking into an interview.

Be the person who gets what the job is about, what the company stands for, and what they're trying to accomplish. This comes with doing your research and understanding what problem they need the new person in this role to help solve.

Always indicate you want the job you're interviewing for by coming out and saying so.

However, if you don't really want the job and you're just interviewing to gain interview practice, this is an unethical practice (just like the one on the interviewer's part in my personal example above), and therefore you shouldn't be there.

This may sound harsh, but as you saw, interviewers can be harsh about very small things. I'm trying to help you get into the mind of the interviewer so you can be successful in your next job interview!

How NOT to overreact (20:26)

Even if you don't get the job offer, you never know what still may come of your experience. Here, because this candidate showed such a positive attitude, another door has been opened to him. The interviewers are setting him up for an interview with another company they think he'll be a good fit for.

A friend of mine interviewed for a job and didn't get the offer. Six weeks later, she got a call from the company asking if she was still interested in the job because the person they originally hired didn't work out.

Things like this happen all the time which is why it's important to stay positive, send your thank you notes after your interviews, and be gracious even when rejected. You never know how things might turn around down the road.

More job interview tips

Based on the little edited snippets we saw of the actual interview, they hired the candidate I would've hired. However, in episode 2, they chose a different candidate than the one I would've chosen. Can you figure out why, based on what you learned above? Watch here and let me know!

For more interview preparation tips, check out the video guides in the Steps to Acing the Interview and

Reducing Your Interview Anxiety on-demand program.

Chapter 11: Identify An Effective Routine

When preparing for an exam, it is important that you are comfortable where you are and that you are not troubled by anything you are not familiar with. As such, an effective study routine would be something that you need to have, if only to ensure that your brain is at optimal level to absorb and process ideas.

Start by identifying the things that you will need. Do you have your notes ready? How about your books? Do you have to use materials from the library for reinforcement of lessons? Do you need the Internet for research? Do you have sample exams you can use for reference? Do you have your pad and pencil ready? Organize your stuff so that you have everything you need ready and within easy reach.

Most people only get down to their notes a day or two before the exam. While this is perfectly understandable, it nonetheless forces the brain to take in concepts more than it can. The result? Panic and stress. These are definitely not a good thing because they only serve to cloud your rational thinking and make you lose your concentration, and in the process affect the way you take the exam -- for the worse.

That idea about people working better under stress? There is a hint of truth to that, although when you think about it, the chances of screwing up are actually higher if you are working under intense conditions within a limited timeframe. So it is still better to set a manageable and completely workable timetable to allow you to better prepare for an exam. Identify the points you need to focus on, the things you need to revise, the stuff you need to read, and other resources to help you out. Do not cram. Doing so often yields either sloppy work or an incoherent understanding of concepts.

Where you study also plays a huge role in how you fare in exams. Start where you normally stay to sort through your notes and other review materials. Most students do so within the comfort of their own rooms. Not only does your own room provide a semblance of privacy, it is also a place that you are very comfortable in and very familiar with. This comfort comes in very handy, especially when you need some quiet and cozy time to study concepts that need multiple re-reading. But therein lies its biggest disadvantage, too: since you have your computer and bed nearby, it is very tempting to be diverted to other things, such as taking a nap or talking to friends online.

The library is a place most students visit to review their studies. The much-needed quiet and the easy availability of reference materials make it very conducive for studying. The library serves as a great spot for those wanting to concentrate on their notes without being distracted unnecessarily. Other places you can go to review or else read are cafes and parks.

Take some time to also consider the time of the day you normally study. Some people are night owls who take advantage of the quiet surroundings during evenings to get down to the business of reviewing for their exams. This makes sense because with almost all people asleep, you get to have little distractions, if at all, so you can concentrate better on what you are doing. Meanwhile, others review for their exams during mornings when their brain is at its most alert. Others do it later in the day when they have finished some of the tasks they have set out to do. Regardless, pick the time of the day that works best for you and stick to it.

Indeed, you need to create an effective routine for studying in order for you to get well-adjusted to factors like the place where you will spend time reviewing and the time of day that you will buckle down to work. When you all these organized down to a T, then reviewing for exams becomes easier and a much pleasant experience.

Chapter 12: Social Anxiety

Regrettably, for some of us, social anxiety has become a real problem and this can stop us interacting effectively socially.

What is social anxiety and how can you recognize if you are a sufferer? Symptoms can be both mental and physical and can often be traced back to childhood experiences. It can make us so scared of being adversely judged by others, that we shun socializing altogether whenever possible and when forced into situations, socially and professionally, can find the symptoms debilitating and paralyzing.

Social anxiety is the third most common mental health problem in America and affects up to 7% of the population at any one time. The condition is chronic, which means it will not go away by itself and needs treatment. Sufferers are often seen by others as being shy and withdrawn, maybe aloof and disinterested. Quite often, however, this is not the case at all.

Sufferers want to make friends and be included in group activities but they do not know how to do it and their lives become a hazardous path when they are put into situations in which they struggle to cope.

There can be a number of triggers which will send sufferers into a panic:

Introductions, especially to authority figures

Being teased or criticized

Public speaking, even to small groups

Eating or drinking in public

Being the center of attention

Entering a room full of people, even if they know them

Answering or speaking on the telephone

Interviews or other formal situations

Being watched or observed when performing a task

Going round the table in a group situation and having to say something

Physical symptoms can include:

Blushing

Stammering

Avoiding looking people in the eyes

Looking down

Hesitating when conversing because they don't know what to say

Swallowing hard

Emotional symptoms:

Irrational fear

Racing heart

Sweating

Tics

Nervousness, e.g. spilling/dropping things

Hands shaking

Dry mouth

Shaking

Feelings of inferiority

Embarrassment

Humiliation

Depression

Self-consciousness

Feelings of inadequacy – 'I can't do that'

Short of breath

Social anxiety is the third prevalent mental health problem after depression and alcoholism. It can exist in just one area of a person's life or it can spread across the board into all areas.

Most sufferers know that their fears are irrational but feel helpless to help themselves. They know that their fears are not based in fact and it is important for sufferers to seek help. CBT – Cognitive Behavior Therapy is an effective way of treating this condition. This helps to change neural pathways and change the way in which sufferers think and feel. It is important to remember that everyone is unique and we will all respond differently.

It is also important to mention that there is a shortage of treatment facilities and should you be lucky enough to find one, you should make it a priority checking out their credentials. Try and find a therapist who is simpatico with you. Saying this, you can carry out very productive techniques yourself, which we will discuss in the next chapter.

Chapter 13: Simple Techniques

We explained to you before that your choice of place to meditate and the time you spend on it is up to you, but there are techniques that can help you a lot with your meditation practice. For example, you will meditate better when you have a clear mind and the breathing that people like Buddhist monks use is particularly deep because it takes a lot of discipline and they believe that this discipline needs to be regulated in some way. In this chapter, we deal with techniques that will help you to get more out of your meditation. The fact that you have already started is great, but perhaps you want to take it a step further than that.

Breathing Techniques

Sit in a comfortable position with your back straight. Posture matters because it helps the air flow. Bow your head a little. This also helps because you are opening up the airways and making it easier to breathe. Breathe in and as you do so, count to 8 and feel the air going down to your upper abdomen. Usually we lightly breathe and it only goes as far as the top of the lungs. Hold the breath for a moment and then breathe out to the count of 10. What you are doing is breathing out longer than you are breathing in and if you get this type of breathing into a rhythm, you will find that you benefit almost straight away because it helps you to be able to meditate in a much calmer way. What you are doing by breathing out for longer is letting out excess stale oxygen from your body and so naturally you will breathe better.

Now try meditating by simply thinking of nothing except the breathing. Breathe in to the count of 8, feel the air going down inside you, and then breathe out to count of ten. Breathe in to the count of 8, feel the air entering your body, breathe out to the count of 10.

This is literally what Buddhist monks do when they meditate but by taking your mind off all the thoughts of the day, you are allowing your mind the clarity that you seek. You are letting go of thoughts. Don't make it a big deal if a thought comes into your mind, but imagine it like a big puff of smoke. it's there one moment and then it's gone! Letting go of thoughts is a little bit hard to start off with but when you practice doing it, you will find it so useful in your everyday life because you will be able to do it almost at will.

Alternate Nostril Breathing

Want a rush of air that helps you to concentrate in a meeting. Why not try this. You may have to lock yourself away from the world for a moment, but it's worth it. Hold your thumb over your right nostril and breathe in through the left nostril. Then switch your thumb over to the left nostril and breathe out of the right nostril. If you do this half a dozen times and make the breath a deep one, just like we used above, this helps you to air out the mind so that you are sharper and your mind is clearer for the meeting. This is something that is practiced by Indian practitioners but it's great for upping your energy levels and can be used at any time that you wish to increase your concentration.

Finding Inner Peace

I think that an exercise in finding your inner peace is a very good one because you can use this when you find that the world is getting on top of you. If you find that the world is getting you down, find a quiet place to sit down away from people. In this place, meditate on something that you can see. It could be a flower or it could be an inspirational picture. Carry a postcard on you that you can use for this. As you look at the chosen object, breathe in to the count of 8 and out to the count of 10 and try to let all other thoughts out of your mind.

It is actually quite hard to think of nothing at all, which is why we suggest that you meditate on a given object. The Buddhist altars in temples are not used for worship. They are used to give the monks something to concentrate on that inspires them. That's why they are such colorful places and really do inspire people. Thus, whatever you choose as your inspiration, you should concentrate on it and nothing else.

If you can keep this up for about 10 minutes, you will find that all of your troubles melt into the background and that you are able to get on with life without having them weigh so heavily upon you. This is a good exercise for lunchtime after a hectic morning at work or can be used to help you to regain your composure after you have been confronted by someone. Step away. Meditate on something inspirational and when you go back to the situation, you will find that your calmness of mind will help you to sort out whatever the problem is without any more friction.

Chapter 14: Learn To Take Control Of

Your Thought

On the off chance that you need to be progressively social what you have to do is to figure out how to take control of your negative idea. You might be in get-together you may feel tense this is because of negative idea in your psyche, what you have to do is to change believed that make you tense to a positive idea. For instance your hand can be shaking openly, this is because of negative idea and negative ideas are ground-breaking since they can influence the mind with the goal that you will trust the idea. What you have to do is to change the negative idea to the idea you want; similarly as negative idea is amazing positive idea are more powerful. Keep at the top of the priority list that your mind thinks all that it hears over and again, particularly in the event that you are stating it. On the off chance that you say, "I CAN'T do that" your mind trusts you, and makes it happen. Right now, you are not ready.

In any case, that doesn't mean we are stuck in our on edge. You can start to change your old silly considerations and convictions by dispensing with the huge, striking, outright words from your self-talk. What you say to yourself more than once is accepted by the cerebrum. In the event that the cerebrum trusts it, it will be valid for you. Whatever you unequivocally accept about yourself comes true. If we utilize this self-talk, our cerebrum hears and trusts each word we say, and after that gets it going. In the event that we trust we can't make an introduction, we can't make an introduction. In the event that we trust we'll never show signs of improvement, we'll never show signs of improvement, except if we figure out how to turn the tables on the idea and supplant our old silly musings and convictions into new judicious considerations and convictions.

The initial phase in turning the tables on the contemplation is to get the enormous, striking silly supreme words and dispose of them from your discourse (your self-talk). This will start to have any kind of effect in the event that you keep your mind open to new clarifications and new choices for why you may be restless. Take out supreme words and keep your mind open.

Chapter 15: Effective Anti-Anxiety

Vitamin, Mineral And Amino Acid

Supplements

When it comes to dealing with anxiety, it would be best to include some of the most effective anti-anxiety vitamins and minerals in your treatment plan. The following are just some of the most effective vitamins and minerals that you should consider incorporating in your treatment plan if you want to deal with anxiety the natural way:

Vitamin B Complex

Excessive fatigue and low energy are two of the major causes of high-stress levels, irritability, and anxiety. In this case, you need B-vitamins that are popular for maintaining high energy levels and boosting cognitive performance. A Vitamin B complex supplement is a major help not only in keeping your energy high but also in lowering your stress levels and preventing anxiety.

Supplementing with this vitamin can even lessen your depressed feelings and personal strain when you are in a high-stress situation. It can also make you feel calm and stable. If you wish to feel more relaxed especially when dealing with a situation that triggers your anxiety, then it would be best to supplement with a Vitamin B complex.

What's good about B-complex vitamins is that they already contain all of the B-vitamins you need, including thiamine (B1), riboflavin (B2), niacin (B3), pantothenic acid (B5), pyridoxine (B6), biotin (B7), inositol (B8), folic acid (B9, and cobalamin (B12). Each of the mentioned B vitamins can affect your body in a different way. As a whole, though, you can expect them to lessen your feelings of anxiety significantly.

Vitamins C and E

It should be noted that your body is prone to undergoing oxidation, a chemical process caused by the release of oxygen as well as molecules known as free radicals. While your body is designed to tolerate oxidation, it is still important to note that it can only do so in small amounts. A high level of free radicals and oxidative stress, therefore, can damage your cells.

Oxidative stress, on the other hand, can lead to anxiety. You can counter these negative effects of oxidative stress and free radicals by taking vitamins rich in antioxidants, like Vitamins C and E. You will notice a significant reduction in your anxiety and panic attacks if you start taking these vitamins.

Magnesium

Magnesium plays several vital roles in your body. If you have problems with anxiety, then it would be best for you to take a magnesium supplement. It is because this mineral works in relaxing your muscles and calming your nervous system. Magnesium also aids in regulating the hormones necessary for promoting relaxation and calming your brain. You can use it to deal with not only anxiety but also muscle spasms and aches, sleeping difficulties, and poor digestion.

When planning to take magnesium, make it a point to look for those forms found in chloride, chelate, and citrate. It is mainly because your body can absorb the mentioned forms better. Just make sure that you begin with smaller doses of magnesium supplement while you are still figuring out the most effective and the safest dose for you. It is because excessive intake of it might also lead to diarrhea.

5-hydroxytryptophan (5-HTP)

Taking a 5-HTP supplement, which is a synthesized version of tryptophan, an essential amino acid for regulating mood, can be a great help in dealing with several issues linked to anxiety, such as headaches, moodiness, and sleeping difficulties. What is good about 5-HTP is that it can also elevate your serotonin level.

Serotonin is known as a calming neurotransmitter, which works in transmitting signals between your nerve cells while altering your brain functions designed to regulate your sleep patterns and mood. 5-HTP can also reduce anxiety significantly because it has calming effects. Just make sure that you avoid taking it together with any anti-depressant or anti-anxiety medications prescribed by your doctor.

Gamma Aminobutyric Acid (GABA)

You can also take advantage of the power of GABA, an amino acid, which plays a major role in reducing anxiety in your nervous system. What is good about GABA is that it relaxes your muscles. You can use it not only in relieving anxiety but also in dealing with other issues, like PMS, insomnia, high blood pressure, pain, and ADHD.

Another benefit of GABA is that it works as an inhibitory neurotransmitter, which has sedative effects, allowing it to calm anxiety and regulate nerve cells. You can also easily access GABA supplements in any vitamin or health food store in your locality. Alternatively, you can take Valerian root, which also works in naturally increasing the level of GABA in your brain and calming anxiety. Check out this vegetarian product: Driftoff Premium Sleep Aid.

Iron

Iron is also a huge help for anxiety sufferers because of the role that it plays in synthesizing serotonin. Also, take note that having iron deficiency can cause anemia, which can also lead to weakness, depression, fatigue, and panic and anxiety attacks.

Make sure, however, that before you take an iron supplement, you consult your doctor and ask him to measure the level of iron within your body through a laboratory testing. This will help ensure that you will be taking the safest and the most appropriate dosage for you.

Chapter 16: Living Without Stress

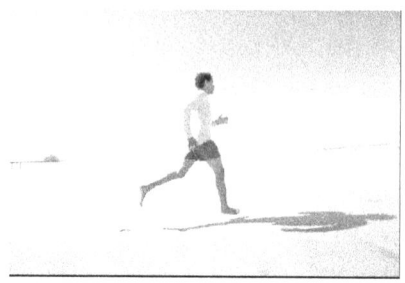

Now that you know what stress is and you have already identified what are the main reasons responsible for causing you stress, is time to start doing some practical measures to help you deal with it.

There are two types of mechanisms used to handle stress. The first one is defensive, characterized by the subconscious, the person distorts the reality in the hope that the situation will change naturally. This posture brings bad results, since it starts to find "acceptable" reasons for our improper behavior. The second is a conscious adaptation mechanism that allows you to change your attitude and learn to foresee your problems. There are four main approaches to deal with stress:

Change the situation, which may require important decisions, such as moving in to a new house, or simple things like changing some of your lamps for better lighting.

Increase your capacity to deal with the situation, which means learning new techniques, such as assertiveness and relaxation techniques.

Change the perspective on the situation, which encourages you to see differently the range of pressures and threats and turn them into challenges.

Change your behavior, change your routine, slow down, do exercise, cut in alcohol and improve your diet.

Exercise

Most people don't do exercise on a daily basis and feels that they are not in shape, the result of that is stress.

The inactivity is bad for your health, causes your metabolism to decrease, make you gain weight, causes high blood pressure and puts your cardiovascular system at risk. The muscles (hearth included), don't work effectively and, gradually, the person becomes more lethargic and tired, starting the vicious cycle. Depression starts to rise, the sexual appetite decreases, joints become stiff and the feeling of poor health grows. These persons avoid physical activities and retract mentally and physically.

Practicing exercise regularly is one of the main keys to remove stress from your life. When you do exercise you burn the excessive adrenalin that is accumulated in your body, making your body more relaxed which then makes your mind more relaxed.

Some sports that are non-competitive and can be beneficial to you are:

Cycling

Marching/running

Swimming

Enjoy the sport and do not focus on the competitive aspect. Your purpose is to have fun and not fight to win or compel to achieve impossible goals.

One important thing when practicing sport is knowing what to eat before and after your exercises and have a good diet plan. How you eat is crucial to have a free stress life. A diverse diet is essential for good health. Always prefer food with high vitamin content, essential fatty acids, antioxidants or unrefined carbohydrate.

Bread

Pasta

Fish

Olive oil

Fresh fruit

Vegetables

Nuts

Yogurt

Fresh vegetables

Garlic

Keep always in mind that there is no such thing as healthy food if you eat too much.

Stress at Work

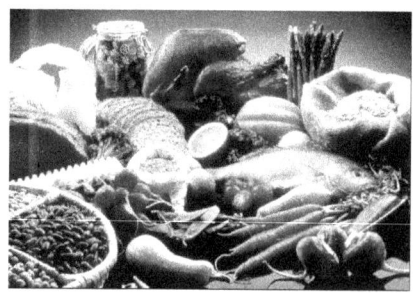

If you know that your work is the reason of your stress, you need to find out what the causes are. Before taking any measures to improve your work environment, you need to identify the problem. Your stress can be caused by many reasons:

Profession intrinsic problems - working conditions, travel, noise or heat.

Career problems - promotions, threat of dismissal, low salary and status.

Problems caused by the organization - control, supervision, poor communication.

Interpersonal relationship problems - friction with others, with superiors, harassment, discrimination based on race, gender or age.

To remove stress that is caused by your job can become quite difficult if the source of your problems is in the organization of your corporation. In that case, as an isolated individual, there is little you can do, but if you discuss these problems with your group maybe you can achieve better results.

If you believe that the main source of your stress is coming from you (due to the fact how you face your job and your coworkers) the solutions are in range. You have to question yourself, so you can decide if you need to change your behavior, work conditions or your job. Here are some questions that you need to answer in order to know what kind of action you need to take:

What do you think about your job? Do you love it or do you hate it?

Do you feel that change of career is a threat or a great challenge?

Do you have de financial resources to do an internship or go back to college?

Do you feel outdated?

Are you able to talk to your boss or professional counselor and explain your problem?

Can you negotiate a flexible work schedule?

Are there alternatives in your company for a work that is less stressful?

Do you know how to be assertive?

You may notice by now that you might not have all the answers for these questions. But by now you have understood that dealing with stress is a complex issue that involves body and mind. The answers are perfectly within your reach.

Maintaining the job that causes you stress may be the only option for you. If that is the case, you need to adapt to the situations. You need to be capable to communicate with others. Dealing with other people in your workspace imply that you have to communicate with people from different levels in your company's hierarchy. The relationships at any level can become quite ambiguous for many reasons, internal policy, misinformation and resentment due to differences in hierarchy, generating several barriers to communication:

Socio-cultural differences - clothes, language, values, age, origin, ethnicity and gender.

Lack of reception of information by the recipient - is too busy, tired or confused, doesn't value the information, have difficulty understanding the message.

Negative attitude of the receiver - had previous bad experiences, do not trust the source, resents authority, depreciates the issuer, hates value judgment.

Mixed Messages - inconsistency in information, different people saying different things, circulation of rumors.

The way that you are treated and the way you treat others can have negative or positive consequences. An authoritarian behavior can both produce obedience because the person feels safe, as rebellion, because the recipient feels that there was no discussion. A paternalistic style can make young and vulnerable people feel protected, but it doesn't encourages independent thinking. A permissive style allows people to develop their own solutions and take on that responsibility, but also creates the danger of opting for easy solutions and disinterested postures. A democratic style provides an exchange of opinions in both directions, as well as incentive awakening of views and strong reasons for disagreement.

If you are unemployed, keep in mind that your situation affects you and your family and friends. The initial reaction to the dismissal includes feelings of rejection, anger, despair, fear, loss, low self-esteem and jealousy. You family and friends will be worried, and don't know what they can say to you that won't bring back bad feelings. Your first priorities would be your financial situation and finding a new job, but, you can look at this situation with a positive perspective.

Use the time you have to reflect about your life, recharge your batteries, identify your resources, plan your time and enjoy the free time you have to rest and relax. If your previous job was stressful, try to look at this situation as an opportunity to find something better, and don't feel guilty for enjoying this time.

Chapter 17: Benefits Of Decluttering Your

Mind

One of the most prominent reasons you want to declutter your mind is because it already is playing a negative role in your life. You may be experiencing its effect right now and may want to do something about it.

Most of the available resources we find online and in print when we look for help point out to dealing with the effects of a cluttered mind. This is just like traditional medicine nowadays which uses treatment to deal with the symptoms, and not with what is causing the symptoms. Self-help books easily tend to dismiss and overlook what is causing the symptoms such as stress, anxiety, unhappiness and so on, and focus on the effects and how to treat it. If you feel stressed, try to work out more, if you feel tired, try to improve your diet, and if you feel miserable, make new friends.

All these pieces of advice have a valid point. But in the end, if you look carefully at the bigger picture, you have to admit that something is missing. No matter how hard you try and succeed in tackling the symptoms that are derived from a cluttered mind, you will need to address the main issue you are facing eventually. Your mind is slowly and steadily becoming your enemy – the cluttering creeps in, step by step, and only by realizing and reversing this process will you be able to put an end to this spiral of unhappiness.

Imagine a mind completely overtaken by fears, stress, worries, anxiety and bad memories. Have you ever thought how much can be accomplished by freeing up the space occupied by these destructive cobwebs? Can you imagine how much freeing up all that blocked mental space can make way for new ideas, feelings, and perspective? Can you imagine the freshness and positivity with which you can live simply by eliminating damaging mental clutter?

Ask yourself this very important question. Are you truly focused on the present in a valuable and meaningful manner? Or do you simply exist, while being preoccupied with thoughts related to completing an assignment before the deadline or replying to an email or thinking about where you should organize your birthday bash? Are you only thinking about your past actions and contemplating the future while totally skipping the joy of being in the present?

Knowingly or unknowingly, all of us inflict upon ourselves a mind filled with chaos, stress, and clutter due to everyday responsibilities. This makes it challenging for us to seek the calm or peace that fills our mind with positivity.

Decluttering isn't simply related to your home or work desk. It starts with our minds; unlike cleaning cupboards, bookshelves and desks, it involves clearing the chaos of negative thoughts and emotions to make way for more productive/constructive ideas and emotions. Unlike a spring-cleaning session, you can't just dump stuff you don't need in a huge donation box and give it away. You have to work every day to clear the mental cobwebs, one at a time until the mind is clean to absorb and retain more positive thoughts.

A clear mind leads to clear thoughts, clear actions, and a clear life. Think of your mind as an inbox, albeit without the technological finesse of sorting junk mail from value adding stuff. This is exactly what makes it so challenging. You have to pick up and sort the stuff yourself to get rid of things (thoughts) that no longer hold relevance or value in your life or those that prevent you from leading a more enriched and rewarding life.

There is plenty of everyday mental junk that doesn't contribute to nourishing the mind in today's fast-paced, technologically slick world. We are being fed with an overdose of "information" that we may not really need. When you input any new information in the brain, it consumes valuable space. Think about it. Your mental resources aren't limitless. When you keep accepting and absorbing new pieces of information, you're cramming it all uncomfortably into a compact space. And lo and behold, if you don't take timely action, you'll end up kicking out the valuable information for the junk stuff. Makes sense?

What happens when we keep buying clothes and accessories we don't really need? We keep shoving them into the wardrobe until they take up all the available space and start tumbling out. The wardrobe door doesn't even shut properly now. You realize there's no place to add new stuff that you really need. What's the best approach? Ta-da, get rid of the unwanted stuff that you don't use with an online or garage sale. It's pretty much the same with mental clutter, only no one's going to buy your clutter. You simply have to find different ways to eliminate it forever.

These disturbing thoughts, distractions, and mental clutter get in the way of helping us perform tasks in a focused manner. Can two objects occupy the exact same available space within your house? No, unless you messily place them one above the other (thus making it challenging to access both). Similarly, two different thoughts can't occupy the exact given space in your mind (again it isn't a limitless resource).

Mental clutter takes us away from the present; out of all the valuable stuff we are working on (or want to focus on). Think about what happens if the mental space is completely freed up only with constructive, valuable and productive thoughts that focus on the present? Think about how much you would benefit simply by staying in the present.

Consider this: modern everyday technology (which was supposed to make our lives easier) has come with inbuilt stress inducers. On an average, a person today receives five times more information that an individual in 1986. Also, almost all the news and insights making their way into your mind is negative (yes because that sells and gets attention).

There are so many worldwide stressors to deal with – the high cost of living, employment issues, soaring cancer rates, global warming, rising crime levels, terrorism and more. Now add your own bunch of stress, sleep problems, anxiety issues to this, and boom that's so much mental clutter to deal with.

When it comes to physical clutter, we simply pile it up and get rid of it to lead a more serene, simple and enriched life.

How about the mental chaos that overtakes our mind and clouds our vision each second of the day? Can you do a mental clean up to clear out the dust and cobwebs? Yes, it is possible (a thousand times over) if you have the sheer resolve to eliminate all the dirt and dust in the corners of your mind to make way for more positive, productive, peaceful and goal-oriented thoughts.

So, how does one declutter mentally? What are the various techniques, ideas, and strategies for practicing mental spring cleaning?

The benefits derived from dealing with the cause rather than the effects are huge.

It is hard not to notice that many of us who try to engage in dealing with problems we're facing in our day-to-day life have limited amounts of energy to spend. We all have to be productive, stay healthy, and take care of others who rely on us for their well-being; at the same time, we have a job or are searching for a job, we are part of a family or a relationship, and we have our dreams, desires, and needs.

The obvious question arises: is it worth fighting to deal with our own problems in such a way that we spend a great deal of time and resources? Does this struggle end eventually? Are we being efficient?

I'm afraid the honest answer is not a positive one.

When we approach an issue that is causing distress by tackling the issue itself, not only do we lose perspective, but we enter a merry-go-round that takes up a lot of effort and energy and gives us the illusion that we are actually advancing towards our goals. After we deal with social anxiety by making new friends, the next issue presents itself, for we've spent a lot of money and time and now we feel insecure and stressed over our costs for day-to-day living. If we work more to cover those new expenses, we end up stressed, tired, unable to maintain the relationships we just developed, and hence we get a new form of social anxiety. And even worse, we feel disappointed, and we blame ourselves for that.

We simply don't know it could be done with little effort. We have no idea that we stand close to the solution, for we are not examining the correct obstacles. For now, keep in mind that there is hardly anyone who can do this on his or her own. Knowledge is power, but at the same time, knowledge is shared and accumulated not as limited individuals, but as a collective mind that constantly improves.

For now, you already feel the answer to the "Why declutter your mind?" question. So, let's engage in building up the whole perspective.

You have the right to a peaceful life, and for this, you need to get rid of your mental clutter. Decluttering is essential to leading a fulfilling life. You cannot enjoy or see the colors of life due to your mental clutter.

Decluttering can be beneficial for you in numerous ways. It also can be attained in numerous ways.

Better Quality of Life

Your thoughts shape the way you live. They shape your interactions and relations. Thoughts even shape your perspective about how you look at life. How will a person view himself and everyone around if he or she isn't able to look clearly through his/her scattered thoughts? Such a person will only see negativity and hatred, his/her relationships will get strained, and he/she won't be able to look at the brighter side of things. However, if you can get rid of all the tangled thoughts, you are trying to open the knots of your mind. When you feel healthy mentally, you will feel fresh and physically healthy as well. All this will improve your quality of life; it will open doors for you. You will be able to form a positive image and ultimately with the decluttering, the quality of your life will improve.

You are your judge. You need to find out who the culprit of your scattered and misty thoughts is. Make a list of the things that affect your mental health and try to get rid of those things. Make efforts to have an organized lifestyle, focus more and prioritize all the tasks in your life. Don't stress out about every little thing, loosen up and try to take things easy. Look at the positivity around you and get rid of the negativity. Make all the possible efforts to declutter your mind. Your mind can shape your life so don't let it get overshadowed by negativity. You are your thoughts so don't let them get polluted by the negative things around you.

Improves Relationship Skills

When you are lost in your thoughts, you often fail to concentrate on the well-being of your relationships. Mental clutter doesn't allow you to step out of yourself. The clutter in your mind strangles you, and eventually your relationships get strained. Decluttering helps to improve your relationships. Once you are in a better state of mind where you don't have to worry about every tiny thing, you get the space to focus on your relationships in a positive way. You will put in an effort to improve your relationship skills. Relationships are built on efforts, sacrifices, and compromises, and these can only be made when you have a relaxed state of mind. You can only put effort into a relationship when you have made enough effort to declutter your mind and have succeeded in it. Strong relationships cannot be built without peace of mind, so decluttering is necessary for a strong foundation of relations and it inevitably leads to the improvement of relationship skills.

Promotes Good Health

Mental health is of the utmost importance. That can only be achieved by being physically healthy. The vast majority of people often ignore this fact. People ignore their mental well-being, and all the scattered thoughts start piling up in their minds. After some time, it becomes so severe that even their physical health starts being affected. To avoid being a part of such a situation, it is advised to make an effort that can help you clear your mental clutter. Mental clutter can lead to numerous mental issues such as anxiety, depression, fear, and anxiousness. Work on yourself as you need yourself the most. Work for your mental well-being. It will not only keep you safe from mental issues, but you will also feel physically healthy.

Health should be your priority, and you need to make an effort to look after yourself.

Helps with Anxiety

Clutter leads to the formation of multiple thoughts. You tend to overthink every little problem, and this eventually leads to anxiety. A permanent state of anxiety isn't right in any aspect of your life. This can lead to strained relationships, professional issues, depression, and anxiousness. Don't let these negative emotions overpower you. Make way for the positivity around you. Once you have embarked on the journey to mentally declutter, you will feel relaxed. You won't panic as much as you do right now and the timespan of anxiety will shorten. When the knots in your mind become untied, the clutter will be cleared. There won't be anything left on which anxiety can feed on, and you will eventually get rid of it. Reducing anxiety is one of the most important benefits of mental decluttering, and it has the power to change your life.

Improves Decision-Making Skills

You will often find yourself in a situation where you are unable to make a decision, and this isn't due to any apparent reason. It's just like you cannot bring yourself to come to a conclusion. All the thoughts get so entangled that you are unable to focus on a single thought. The mental clutter hinders your ability to make a decision. To make a decision, a clear state of mind is required. A decision made with peace of mind allows for the decision, in most cases, to be the right one and not one made on hasty grounds. Decluttering leads to a peaceful state of mind. It helps you to focus on your surroundings and thoughts without being anxious. Most importantly, timely decisions ensure you make wise decisions.

Relieve Stress

The world has become so chaotic and society so demanding that every other person around you is feeling stressed. People from the age of 18-28 are said to be the most stressed. Why is that so? The reason for this is because everyone is trying to do many things at a single time. The thoughts aren't focused. All this leads to anxiety as you have become presumptuous about other people. To fit the set norms of society is even adding more stress. What do you do then? Try to streamline your thoughts, prioritize your goals, organize and try to focus more, and in a better way. The more you declutter your mind, the more you will feel relieved. When you learn to organize and focus, you won't panic, and ultimately it will save you from all the stress that you used to go through earlier.

Chapter 18: Make Yourself A Priority

"You can search the entire universe, and not find a single being more worthy of love than you."

– Buddha

I finally woke up to the truth, "if it's to be, it's up to me." I do not recall who said it, but I memorized the words and added them to my ongoing list of mantras. "If it's to be, it's up to me." . . . . . . repeated over and over.

"Whatever you can do or dream you can, begin it. Boldness has genius, power and magic in it!" – Johann Wolfgang von Goethe (1749-1832), German Poet, Playwright, Novelist.

Okay Johann Wolfgang von Goethe, you're on!

For starters, I read every book on personal development I could get my hands on, took a sabbatical from my daily routine and ruthlessly questioned my spirituality and challenged my very existence.

My search led me to a seminar in Hawaii led by Tony Robbins, motivation speaker, seminar leader, and author of "Unlimited Power." I learned that I can choose my power. If I can't, I must; if I must, I will.

Tony Robbins is a master at helping people see through their self-imposed limitations, to think and act outside the box, to let their own magnificence shine through the clouds of doubt. After two weeks of high intensity learning, preparations were made for the final test of courage, the Fire Walk, which I participated in. More about that later.

I also did a tandem jump with a tandem master. I have always been fearful of heights, but I was empowered by the seminar and bravely jumped from an airplane flying at approximately 8,000 feet on a cloudless and calm morning.

I had finally experienced freedom from fear and self-doubt! And would I find the courage and tenacity of heart to succeed; yes, I proved it!

Also at the seminar I met and was deeply moved by the sincerity of Dr. Robert Cialdini, President of Influence at Work (IAW), Arizona State University Regent's Professor Emeritus of Psychology and Marketing, a New York Best Selling Business Author. From him I learned that the principles and techniques of persuasion can be learned by everyone and with practice, we become one with it. It served me well as I charted my way through the maze of co-worker and client personalities I encountered each day. It helped me once again be a part of society after months of self-imposed isolation. My confidence soared!

I became a Dr. Deepak Chopra "groupie" and followed him from his first appearance in Milwaukee, Wisconsin to Atlanta, Georgia; Boston, Massachusetts, and San Diego, California. Dr. Chopra, speaker and a prominent Alternative Medicine advocate, is one of the great leaders in the field of mind-body medicine. He is the author of several dozen books, including Ageless Body, Timeless Mind, Quantum Healing, and Perfect Health.

I learned healing comes from within. One effective way to tap into that healing power is by meditation, practiced daily.

I also learned that greed, jealousy, envy, and comparing one's self to others creates disharmony in the melody of life and is the cause of many diseases. I eliminated those elements from my life in order to clearly see my way through the confusion and darkness that once overwhelmed me.

When Dr. Chopra was in Milwaukee, a friend of mine who has been a hairdresser for fifteen years asked for his advice. As a result of standing on her feet all those years, her ankle caused her constant pain and her doctor advised surgery. She felt she needed a second opinion and explained her concerns to Dr. Chopra. His advice was "Meditate, Meditate, Meditate."

Chapter 19: Eating Well

Just as important as moving well and being active is eating well. If you do not eat well then, frankly, you are going to notice the massive limitations that it can have on your quality of life. Failing to eat right when depressed will simply fuel the symptoms.

I get how easy it is to fall into the trap, having done so myself. A bar of chocolate, a movie bag of crisps…it's so easy to do. However, living on a diet of junk food and drinking soft drinks, and alcohol too often, will lead to a slow and sluggish body. It will tend to lead to digestive issues, alongside gaining massive amounts of weight.

This is going to leave you feeling worse generally but is also likely to put you into a position where you hate how you look. This will bring down your self-esteem further and make the climb from the abyss that little bit tougher than it has to be.

Instead of eating all this junk, making a positive change to your diet can be the catalyst to long-term health improvement that you seek. This is very useful for you to make sure that you fully understand the next step–replacing soda with water, chips with vegetables and fast food with home cooked meals is a wonderful step.

Home cooked meals, by the way, are a great way to get yourself active too. You need to get the ingredients and make it yourself, meaning that you have something to occupy your time with and–crucially–something to achieve. Just make sure that you cook for two, because in a depressed state of mine you will likely think the food you have made is horrible!

Avoid drinking too much, as well. Alcohol can lead us down dark paths mentally and can be a long-term problem to deal with later in life. If you start to drink when you feel sad it can amplify that feeling and make you concentrate on the fear, the grievance and the anger that you have built up. This is not healthy and only serves to fuel depression, not fight it.

Additionally, alcohol is full of emptycalories–even a couple of glasses could have you consumingextra calories. Weight gain leads to more poor eating habits to escape the fear, which makes it so much easier to loathe who you are. It's a vicious cycle and one that you need to avoid if you are serious about defeating depression and anxiety.

The diet you live on might not be the sole cause of your depression, but it can be one of the leading players. At the very least, it will make you more active mentally just by eating right. Making this adjustment now is going to make it so much easier for you to begin to make that shift from depressed to fearless. I found that by changing my diet I became more positive in the mind. I noticed a change in how I lived and how I thought. Before long, that positivity spread!

Chapter 20: Your Emotion Can Keep Or

Kill You

God's perfect desire is for you to live long, strong and healthy. But you must know what crucial part your emotions hold in the total well-being of your life.

The truth is that a life that is full of joy and happiness lives longer than those who are angry, depressed and have bitterness.

A merry heart does good, like medicine, But a broken spirit dries the bones.

Proverbs 17:22

Most diseases are associated with bad and wrong emotions. The truth of the matter is that your emotions. The truth of the matter is that your emotion can shorten or prolong your life. Dr Don Colbert says "your heart and your body are more powerfully connected than you know."

Experts have said that when you keep being positive, happy and laughing all time, certain hormones are continually released into your body. These hormones repair damaged cells, create a feeling of well-being. Laughter, they say keeps some vital organs inside you (like liver, lungs, etc) properly massaged to perform their functions. All of these contribute to your living long, strong, and healthy.

God originally created the body to repair itself and remain in health, but when you overload the body with negative emotion and attitude, you destroy its capacity.

STOP THE NEGATIVE THING

Dr. Colbert gave such a tremendous insight into the formation of bad emotions. Wrong emotions develop from wrong thoughts.

1. If you are always critical of people you will end up developing emotions of envy and jealousy.

2. Those always complaining will develop negative emotion of Selfishness and Greed. You become greedy and

selfish.   Once you conquer this habit, you can conquer the emotion.

3.   Those   always   grumbling   and complaining end up with negative emotion of Bitterness and Resentment.

4.   An argumentative habit leads to anger.

5.   A person who always sees the negative side of things will develop a negative   emotion   of   depression, hopelessness and tiredness in his/her soul. They just get tired beyond the physical. They just don't have the energy to face tomorrow.   This   is   when   negative emotions of suicide begin to come.

6.   When you are always taking offense and you are too irritable, you will end up with a negative emotion of resentment. But the Bible says you can change all that, Proverbs 17:22

The Knox translation of the Bible critically says "A cheerful heart makes a quick recovery, it is crushed spirit that wastes a man's frame".

So when you are living with a negative attitude or a negative emotion your frame is wasted. This means sickness and diseases will take over the body. The simple reason is that your immune system is beaten down and is no longer strong enough to resist any disease.

When you become up-beat in your emotion, when you start getting joyful and happy, right hormones are secreted into your body and this brings strength and healing. The joy of the LORD always bring strength.

Then he said to them, "Go your way, eat the fat, drink the sweet, and send portions to those for whom nothing is prepared; for this day is holy to our Lord. Do not sorrow, for the joy of the LORD is your strength."

Nehemiah 8:10

This is God's mandate: dwell in joy all the time.

The church praise and worship time helps you to get well. "Get happy and get well." To be low in spirit is to be sapped of health and strength. Where there is bitterness, resentment, unforgiving, depression and anger, the body is automatically programmed for disease and death. God in His love gave us the Spirit of Joy to live long, strong and healthy.

To console those who mourn in Zion, To give them beauty for ashes, The oil of joy for mourning, The garment of praise for the spirit of heaviness; That they may be called trees of righteousness, The planting of the LORD, that He may be glorified."

Isaiah 61:3

When you begin to enter into the joy of the Lord and put on garment of praise, heaviness will lift, and you can live long, strong and planted for the glory of your God in health not in disease.

NEGATIVE EMOTIONS AFFECT THE HORMONAL AND CHEMICAL RELEASES OF YOUR BODY

Watch those who are always upset, they are always angry, they are always worried. They never have good digestion of their food. The food will ferment and produce toxins instead of digestion because enough hydrochloric acids are not released under the stress of negative emotions. When your food is not properly digested, bloating of stomach, excess gas, heartburn and so forth can start happening. Check out your emotional level. Do not allow stress to accumulate.

Dr. Colbert listed a host of health problems associated with negative emotion. He says hatred and jealousy can lead to high blood pressure, ulcers, migraine headache, cancer and heart disease.

The simple reason is that the body is denied enough release of hormones and chemical balances that will help your body fight diseases.

If your immune system gets suppressed, your body will be open to attack. Negative emotions can kill. Destroy them today. Attack the root-cause now then you will not come under attack.

Emotional pressure can suppress your immunity. Some people store up issues in their heart. They internalize issues so much. They dwell on it and brood over issues.

THE BAD EMOTION OF FEAR AND ANXIETY

When you are gripped with fear or anxiety, your body responds immediately. Fear and anxiety just trigger the excessive release of adrenaline into your body. Expert calls this: "your fight or flight response".

The problem is that if someone is always under fear and anxiety, the adrenaline gland will constantly be under pressure to release adrenaline. This can lead to adrenal exhaustion, extreme fatigue, tension, headache and other disease.

God says you should have nothing to fear.

You are of God, little children, and have overcome them, because He who is in you is greater than he who is in the world.

1 John 4:4

The Lord is already your God, trust in him.

For I am the LORD your God, The Holy One of Israel, your Savior; I gave Egypt for your ransom, Ethiopia and Seba in your place. Since you were precious in My sight, You have been honored, And I have loved you; Therefore I will give men for you, And people for your life. Fear not, for am with you; I will bring your descendants from the east, and gather you from the west; I will say to the north, 'Give them up!' And to the south, 'Do not keep them back!' Bring My sons from afar, and My daughters from the ends of the earth— everyone who is called by My name, Whom I have created for My glory; I have formed him, yes, I have made him."

Isaiah 43:3-7

You may be passing through the fire or deep waters of life. When the Lord is strongly your anchor, faith can be released for a miracle.

ANXIETY CANNOT HELP YOU

Be anxious for nothing, but in everything by prayer and supplication, with thanksgiving, let your requests be made known to God; and the peace of God, which surpasses all understanding, will guard your hearts and minds through Christ Jesus.

Philippians 4:6-7

Let your faith in His Word be strong. Meditate scriptures on God's possibility power.

For with God nothing will be impossible."

Luke 1:37

Jesus said to him, "If you can believe, all things are possible to him who believes."

Mark 9:23

"God is not a man, that He should lie, nor a son of man, that He should repent. Has He said, and will He not do? Or has He spoken, and will He not make it good?

Numbers 23:19

These scriptures will keep you trusting until your miracle is done. Deal with anxiety and fear now. They can destroy. Anger destroys so fast.

Dr. Robert Ellions, a noted Cardiologist, confirms that when "hot reactors" internalize their feelings, it can turn into hostility and range. Then the blood pressure goes up so high.

Anger actually leads to a development of high blood pressure. The person comes under an increased risk of developing heart attack, stroke and other diseases. God has given us a strong warning about anger.

Be angry, and do not sin"; do not let the sun go down on your wrath. Ephesians 4:26

Never dwell on issues for long as to cause you anger. The pain of any situation is as long as you keep the remembrance. Anger is deadly. It is only foolishness to keep getting angry when you know that anger can destroy.

Do not hasten in your spirit to be angry, for anger rests in the bosom of fools.

Ecclesiastes 7:9

DEPRESSION IS DEADLY

Do you wonder why those who didn't plan their retirement well die just so quick in depression most often? Researchers say whenever there is no HEALTHY EMOTIONAL OUT LET, the immune system can be suppressed, and this can actually lead to other diseases including cancer.

If you notice despair in your life, quickly get back to the Word and take in the Word. It encourages your faith when you do that for a while. At such moments locate God's promises and dwell on them.

If you notice bitterness against somebody, instead of allowing it to block your communication with God and destroy your health, get to the person and release it. Positively take it out in love so the anger and bitterness will not destroy you. Jesus tells us not to internalize any issue bothering is. Get across to the person and settle it quick. It will help your health. It will sensitize the environment and keeps everyone in peace.

"Moreover if your brother sins against you, go and tell him his fault between you and him alone. If he hears you, you have gained your brother. But if he will not hear, take with you one or two more, that 'by the mouth of two or three witnesses every word may be established.' And if he refuses to hear them, tell it to the church. But if he refuses even to hear the church, let him be to you like a heathen and a tax collector.

Mathew 18:15-17

Make it up. You may not even be the guilty person but your health is so important to you. So do what He says. Your contact with God is so important so do what God says.

"And whenever you stand praying, if you have anything against anyone, forgive him, that your Father in heaven may also forgive you your trespasses.

Mark 11:25

Release people from your heart by forgiveness. You can forgive.

1.   You will realize that even if you hold it against the person it does not change the circumstance. So then let go.

2.   You can forgive when you change your focus from revenge to love.

When your heart is full of revenge, you can't forgive, but recognize that God had every right not to forgive our sins —but He allowed love to prevail.

 But God demonstrates His own love toward us, in that while we were still sinners, Christ died for us.

Romans 5:8

3. You can ask the Holy Spirit to help you. The love of God is already in your heart — but you need the help of the Holy Spirit, particularly if you are born again, to be able to release love to the unlovable.

4. You can forgive because your health will be jeopardized if you keep offenses in your heart.

5. You can forgive because your relationship with God and man will be jeopardized if you don't forgive.

But you ask can't God understand? Yes He does understand, but He wants you to live long, strong and healthy, that's why He does not want you to store up wrong emotions. You can forgive now.

The issue now is not even the one you hold a grudge against, the issue is that your life is in danger. That is the reason you must learn forgiveness.

YOU CAN CONQUR PRIDE

Recognize that greatness you enjoy came from God.

Every good gift and every perfect gift is from above, and comes down from the Father of lights, with whom there is no variation or shadow of turning

James 1:17

So, why not be humble enough to give thanks to God for where He brought you in life. String appreciation to God will reflect in your healthy living.

When you start appreciating God- you star being joyful in your heart that you are recognizing the source of your blessing, and when you start being joyful, you become health-full

Watch against any wrong emotion. Whether it is fear, anger, bitterness, resentment or pride, they all in one way or the other have effects on your health.

See what pride did to Herod.

So on a set day Herod, arrayed in royal apparel, sat on his throne and gave an oration to them. And the people kept shouting, "The voice of a god and not of a man!" Then immediately an angel of the Lord struck him, because he did not give glory to God. And he was eaten by worms and died.

Acts 12:21-23

We do not have to look for explanations for this. Herod's body gave way. His health just decayed. Pride dethroned and destroys. Run away from them. Think about the type of insanity that came upon King Nebuchadnezzar because of pride.

At the end of the twelve months he was walking about the royal palace of Babylon. The king spoke, saying, "Is not this great Babylon, that I have built for a royal dwelling by my mighty power and for the honor of my majesty?"

While the word was still in the king's mouth, a voice fell from heaven: "King Nebuchadnezzar, to you it is spoken: the kingdom has departed from you! And they shall drive you from men, and your dwelling shall be with the beasts of the field. They shall make you eat grass like oxen; and seven times shall pass over you, until you know that the Most High rules in the kingdom of men, and gives it to whomever He chooses."

Daniel 4:29-32

Nebuchadnezzar became a companion of beasts and an eater of grass because of pride. Never allow pride in your life so that you are not deprived of the things of life.

Chapter 21: Develop The Right Mindset

Your mindset is the set of ideologies, beliefs, suggestions, and opinions you believe in; it governs your life. If you believe in being punctual, you will be punctual and regular in everything you do. If you believe you are not capable of doing something, you will forever nurture this belief and will most likely never fulfill your goals.

Broadly, there are two types of mindsets: a positive and growth mindset, and a negative limiting mindset. You support either a positive mindset or a negative one. If you have a positive mindset, that's great for you because it means you are an optimistic person, who is hopeful and awaits good possibilities and things to come to you.

As opposed to this, if you nurture a negative mindset, every likelihood is that your life is in a miserable state, which makes being mindful a challenge. To embrace mindfulness, you need to build the right mindset and then strengthen it.

Let us now discuss how a negative mindset is damaging to you, how a positive one helps you become mindful and then detail the steps and strategies you can use to build the right mindset.

Negative vs. Positive Mindset

You may have experienced many instances where you felt not good enough to do a certain professional or personal task. For instance, if you look back, you can perhaps remember a time when your boss asked you to lead an important new product marketing campaign.

That responsibility may have made you feel important and even thought that if you carried it out well, you would receive a great promotion. However, you doubted your capabilities and expertise, which caused you to have second thoughts about accepting the offer.

Well, the possibilities are; you did not accept that challenge and missed a valuable opportunity to excel and grow, a decision you regret till date, or you accepted it, but let your lack of self-confidence cloud your rational thinking and skills, which led to a poor job. Observe both scenarios, and you will understand the reason behind both failures: your negative mindset.

In the above instance, since you did not have control over your thoughts, you allowed a negative thought to feel overpowered and brew a concoction of similar thoughts that slowly poisoned you. As a result, you doubted yourself and kept thinking of all the undesirable consequences that may happen if you do the job wrong instead of being mindful, staying in the present, and making the best use of the opportunity.

As opposed to this, if you had believed in yourself and had a positive mindset, you'd have easily combatted the negative thought with a calming, supportive, and optimistic suggestion such as, "Don't worry, you'll do great; just believe in yourself." This suggestion would have helped you focus on the present and enjoy the opportunity that would have brought growth into your life.

This clearly shows how detrimental a negative mindset is to you and your ability to practice mindfulness. The above also illustrates why you need to eliminate a negative mindset from your life.

Here are the different strategies you can employ to replace a negative mindset with a positive one and stay mindful of your everyday life.

Accept Your Negative Thoughts and Listen to Them

To be mindful, you have to learn to acknowledge everything that happens to you and accept it the way it is without judging it. Once you acknowledge it, you then have to look for ways to fix the issue without being critical of it.

Similarly, to shun negative thinking, you first have to acknowledge your negative thoughts and hear what they have to say.

One reason why you cannot move past negative thoughts is not paying attention to them.

To acknowledge your negative thoughts, grab a notebook and a pen and sit somewhere quiet. Practice mindful breathing for five minutes and then focus on all the reasons why you feel stuck in a position or feel miserable at heart. You may come up with ideas and thoughts like, "I have a good job, but I am never my true-self in front of others and try pleasing people because I lack self-belief." "I don't do things I enjoy because I fear if I am my unique self, people will criticize me," "I don't have the nerve to pursue my goal because it is too daunting and I'm not skilled enough to fulfill it," or other similar thoughts.

As they come to you, write these thoughts in your notebook. Stay mindful of a thought as it flows in your mind and read it slowly immediately after writing it in your journal. Once all negative thoughts are out in the open, verbally say "thank you" to yourself for being aware of these thoughts, then write a comforting note that states how appreciative you are of your subconscious mind for making you aware of thkoktgese thoughts that exist in your mind. Intentionally promise yourself to make efforts to calm these thoughts so you can feel better about yourself.

Notice how this suggestion has no critical or analytical words or phrases that have a negative connotation. It simply states that you have accepted those thoughts and your desire to calm them without labeling them unhealthy or pessimistic. This simple suggestion makes you mindful of the negativity inside you and encourages you to manage it calmly and positively.

Replace Negative Thoughts and Beliefs with Positive Ones

Once you acknowledge negative thoughts, replace them with positive ones. Doing that may seem a little difficult at first, especially if you are a people pleaser, lack self-esteem, or the ability to be your true self.

In that case, first, describe who you truly are in a paragraph, and then loudly say, "I wholeheartedly accept myself. I'm proud of myself." Next, build a positive suggestion to calm each negative thought and write this positive thought 20 times while you speak it aloud.

For instance, if a negative thought states, "I hate myself for being a people pleaser," then change this to 'Pleasing people is a kind habit. However, I am now concentrating on pleasing myself and being happy before I please others." Similarly, change different negative thoughts and transform them into happier, healthier ones.

Once you do this, discard the paper full of negativities, and severally re-read the paper full of positive thoughts; consistently do this every day until it becomes a habit. To ensure this happens, use a positive reinforcement, such as a treat or anything nice that makes you feel good for about two weeks each time you practice this every day without fail. In addition, be grateful for what you have so you can build a positive mindset.

Developing Gratitude to Strengthen Mindfulness

Developing gratitude means being thankful for all the little to big blessings in your life and for your life itself. When you are thankful for your life, you acknowledge the many blessings bestowed upon you and become content with what you have in your present life. This keeps your thoughts grounded in the present without giving them a chance to lurk in the past or future because you are pleased with all you have and yourself.

Moreover, being grateful also reinforces a positive mindset. When you look at how nice your house is, or the healthy, nutritious food you eat while many people die from hunger, you stop complaining about the luxury car you do not have or the lacking 72" plasma TV. Instead, you focus on your blessings; this makes you mindful and positive.

To make gratitude an integral part of your life, develop a morning ritual of identifying any five blessings in your life. These could be anything that makes your life comfortable, enjoyable, convenient, and meaningful. If having a laptop, a loving mother, and an air conditioner makes your life better in any way, these could be your blessings. After recognizing your blessings, verbally and literally (in written form) thank the universe for these blessings.

Next to each blessing, write a note about how much it helps you live a better life. To improve mindfulness, gratitude, and positive mindset, do this every day.

In addition, you need to improve your mindfulness practice so you can improve your level of mindfulness and ensure negative influences never bother you again. To do this, you need various tips and strategies.

Chapter 22: Stress Effects Overall

There is no doubt about it; stress has been proven to make you sick. We already know that stress contributes to heart disease; it causes high blood pressure and causes the immune system not to work correctly. It's linked to irritable bowel syndrome, strokes, diabetes, ulcers, joint and muscle pain, miscarriages, alopecia, allergies and early tooth loss.

Have you ever found when stressed you want to sit down and eat a whole pint of ice cream? There is a medical reason for that. It is a hormone, called cortisol that is released when you are stressed, that links you to crave for fats and sugars. Some reach for a candy bar, some ice cream, some pure chocolate.

What makes it worse besides the cravings? It can increase the amounts of fat that your body is storing for you, and it enlarges the size of your fat cells. Who wants that? It will lead to increased risk for high blood pressure, high cholesterol, obesity and the list goes on. I think you get the idea.

If you suffer from severe or chronic stress, your hair can start to fall out, not a little; I mean a LOT. And if your stress is piled on top of anxiety, it can cause you to have a mental disorder that makes people start pulling their hair out.

If you happen to suffer from chronic stress, it can shorten the telomeres, which are protective camps at the ends of chromosomes in your cells, causing you to age more quickly.

Some people are so sensitive to stress that they suffer from seizure-like symptoms. They may stare far off into the distance and go into convulsions when they get into an extremely high-stress situation.

Studies conducted in the United States have already demonstrated that if you remove the stressors that it improves certain aspects of a person's health. Managing your stress has been found to

160

be capable of reducing heart attacks by 75% in those with heart disease. Managing stress and methods of anger management, helped reduce high blood pressure, and for the patients who suffered from chronic tension headaches, it found that by using stress management techniques it allowed the prescribed drugs to be more efficient. The bottom line is that these ailments are made worse by stress.

Dealing with stress can significantly reduce important brain functions like concentration, learning, memory, all of which are ultimately necessary to perform effectively at work.

There are some health effects brought on by stress that is so severe that they are irreversible and some can be fatal.

Chapter 23: Love Yourself

"Your task is not to seek for Love, but merely to seek and find all the barriers within yourself that you have built against it." - Rumi

What is Self-Love?

Self-love means showing compassion to ourselves. You are not to be harsh with yourself and criticize every single thing. We often tend to do that when things don't go quite our way. Every time someone does a task better than us, we often blame ourselves for simply not being perfect.

A human being is made to make mistakes. But berating yourself on them relentlessly can cause serious damage to your self-esteem. The lower your self-esteem goes, the more likely you are to fall into depression and anxiety.

Practicing self-love techniques builds greater self-esteem. Better self-esteem is directly linked to good mental health. Self-compassion brings about these constructive habits.

Optimistic nature.

Lesser depression.

Lesser anxiety.

Putting the stress behind oneself.

We have to realize that mistakes and struggles are part of life. Those imperfections are what reality is. Self-love has some aspects to it, which are:

Humanity: To know you are just human and can make mistakes, but they don't define you.

Kindness: Like you treat the people around you with generosity. Self-kindness means also diverting some of that tenderness to yourself.

Mindfulness: Developing a healthy and non-judging point of view. It is about cultivating an open and curious mindset.

Self-love will give you hope and will help you pursue healthy behaviors in life.

Self-Compassion

Some simple steps for self-compassion are as below:

Recognize when you are giving into a negative state of mind. If anxiety starts to creep up, then it is time to call it out. Acknowledge that these feelings are affecting you. It's better to accept than shut it out completely.

Imagine if your loved one was going through the same thing, what would your reaction be. It won't be harsh and criticizing, will it? You will be kind and caring because you know they don't deserve it.

Rather than blaming yourself for your behavior, try to find an explanation for it and don't judge yourself immediately. Everything is not always black and white. It is our anxiety that tends to make us feel vulnerable and not be comfortable with ourselves and our thoughts. Making mistakes is common, but accepting them and promising to yourself to change for the better, is what real growth is as a person.

We often categorize ourselves to the lowest of the low and put others on the highest stage where they are practically flawless, which, in fact, is not true at all. Most successful people have owned to making great blunders. What they didn't do afterward is let those shortcomings of theirs to put a damper on their accomplishments. They believed in themselves and carried on.

If you have done something horrid, you feel responsible for, then it is not healthy to wallow in it forever. At some point, you have got to get up and think about what can be done to make amends. Those who love will support you, but ultimately it is up to you to make changes for the sake of yourself. You have to take the reins of your own life.

Self-love and Anxiety Disorders

Self-love is being patient and amiable towards yourself so that you can develop healthy habits essential for wellbeing. To find inner peace, it is necessary to practice loving yourself. When you truly love yourself, you can achieve true happiness. How can you be truly happy when on the inside you don't accept yourself?

Loving yourself is not to be translated into egoistic behavior. It is definitely not narcissism. Self-love doesn't mean you stop caring about values and do what you constantly want because that is what makes you happy. It is not built on the feeling of jealousy and envy. Those green monsters are opposite to self-care.

It is a feeling of being worthy of happiness. No matter what you do, you cannot escape your body. So it is better not to make it a prison for yourself. By being honest, accepting, and respectable towards yourself, you are truly allowing yourself to evolve into a better version.

If you don't love yourself how can you extend that feeling towards others?

Techniques of self-love for anxiety

Self-love helps in the portrayal of how you behave and defines your personality. Self-love promotes self-confidence. It can lead you to succeed at work and in your social life. It is one of the best weapons against anxiety. By regularly practicing self-love, you are sure to lead an anxiety free life. Self-love will readily prompt you to make healthier life changes. So by design, a healthy lifestyle keeps you away from anxiety and stress.

Most sensitive people are often prone to anxiety. Realizing that you are not what you feel is the first step to heal. If you feel overwhelmed, then this realization can give you a clear perspective and help you get rid of that feeling.

1. Get to know yourself better and don't be swayed easily by others' opinions of you. People who have self-love don't act in accordance to what others want. If you are in tune with your inner self, you will automatically experience less anxiety.

2.   Surround yourself with people who truly care about your wellbeing. If you realize someone is detrimental for your mental health, then there is no shame in cutting away from that relationship. If you have a positive environment around you, it will help you more with your anxiety.

3.   Practice conscious breathing. As soon as you feel like stress is going to get you and you will get a panic attack, talk positively to yourself. If you are facing a hectic schedule or any situation that makes you nervous, some positive self-talk is a great coping mechanism. Verbally outlay things you need to do and ensure yourself that you will get through it.

4.   Indulge yourself in self-soothing habits, such as running a scented bath or using a calming scent in your house. Put on your favorite show. Get in the comfiest outfit that you can find. Seek warmth, sit by a cozy fireplace.

5.   Enjoy some superfoods. They will impact your blood sugars and energy levels. It will help regulate those. Food

impacts our brain and thus our mood also. Some of these superfoods are below.

Almonds

Chocolate

Berries

6.   There is a phenomenon known as 'Biophilia.' It explains that humans feel calmer and stress-free in nature. So try to connect with earth any way you can and you don't need to be a hiker or climber. You can tend to a small garden or visit the park, etc. Playing with sand also reduces stress so just build a sand castle at the beach.

7.   Acupressure has been practiced throughout centuries and people have documented its advantages. There are two acupuncture points located between the skull and neck. They are said to help with stress and anxiety. This is what you need to do if you want to try it.

Place your thumbs at the top of the neck. It where the neck meets your skull

Apply gentle pressure.

The pressure must not be soft but firm. Keep pressing and throughout it slowly and deeply breathe three times.

After that lazily float your hands in your lap.

Then drop your chin to your chest slowly.

In the end, take a deep breath and smile to top it off.

You have to start with love to get away from negativity. Anxiety triggers negative emotions like a shame for not being able to do things, not being able to handle situations and having a constant fear of anxiety attack. Anxiety is a one step forward two step backward kind of thing. You must have loads of patience. This is real life, not a movie where a single moment tends to make everything better. It is a good place to start your journey, but the real deal is the ride to reach that finish line.

How not loving yourself causes anxiety

When you don't care about your wellbeing, then it is called self-abandonment. It is directly related to anxiety.

Emotional self-abandonment is when you deliberately don't pay attention to how anxiety is making you suffer inside out. Loving yourself emotionally means you have a strong inner bond in place. When things upset you, rather than feeling helpless, you work it out with yourself. Anxiety will struggle to get hold of you if you start to practice true self-love.

Physical self-abandonment happens when we let ourselves go and don't think what is healthy for us. We don't sleep enough, don't drink water enough, or have an unhealthy diet. All of these things, if not resolved, are a one-way ticket to anxiety kingdom. Loving yourself physically means taking care of your diet and health. Health is true wealth after all.

Financial self-abandonment means that either you overspend and regret afterward or you don't spend money at all not even for your basic needs. When you do spend, you want to get the cheapest thing for fulfilling your need. You are not enjoying yourself this way and it can lead to unhappiness. Troubles with money related to debt are one of the biggest causes of stress.

Organized self-abandonment means that your schedule is a mess. You are not organized in your daily life. Being a bit mature and adult-like is helpful. Being organized and following a schedule are keys to success and will make you less prone to anxiety.

Relationship self-abandonment means that in a relationship, it is important that you resolve conflict not by giving in and going along with whatever the other person wants. You have to make them see what you want and then you both have to work on it. If you are constantly putting yourself down just to please others, it will end up doing you and your relationship more harm than good.

Spiritual self-abandonment is when you don't ask your higher power for guidance, wisdom, and love then it is likely that you will end up feeling lonely and depressed. Loving yourself spiritually means to stay in contact with higher power and seek peace within, so you can efficiently fight off anxiety.

Disadvantages of Low Self-Esteem

Low self-esteem is generally caused by not giving any regard to yourself. Having low self-esteem is often linked to anxiety disorders.

Social anxiety disorder

If you have low self-esteem, you are more likely to develop a social anxiety disorder later on. Low self-esteem can make one feel lonely. It highlights more negative aspects of your image to yourself.

Social anxiety disorder's main cause could be pinpointed as having low self-esteem. You built negativity around yourself based on some bad moment that happened. It affects nearly 7% of America's adult population ("What Are Anxiety Disorders?" 2019)[11].

General anxiety disorder

General anxiety disorder is often linked to having low self-esteem. It is a feeling of being unworthy. Self-esteem of a person develops by how they view themselves based on others' reactions towards them. People who are showered with lots of affections by others tend to have high self-esteem. Those who are getting rejected don't have a lot of self-confidence. People with anxiety disorder experience more rejection from their surroundings; some of it is all in their heads though. They will also be loved, but they fail to see it. 2% of the American adult population is affected by this mental health disorder ("What Are Anxiety Disorders?" 2019)[12].

You should evaluate how much people stand by you and how much they neglect you. One important question is how much do they matter to you? If they don't matter to you, then their rejection doesn't hold a lot of meaning. If they are closer ones, then it is usually stress and anxiety that is pushing them away. Seeking therapy for GAD will help you improve your relationships.

People with anxiety and low self-esteem become stuck and inactive. They feel demoralized to perform an action because of all the negative reasons they have conjured in their mind. General anxiety disorder will hinder your ability to take action.

Remember to acknowledge your accomplishments and thinking back to them will give you motivation.

Advantages of self-love

As you get more confident in ourselves, you tend to delay tasks, less in favor of perfection, as you did before. You develop a go-getter attitude that helps you pursue talks more easily.

We don't let failure get us down. We know setbacks are not intended to be mulled over, but to learn from and move on.

We learn to not let criticism get to us. We acknowledge negative feedback, but we don't take it as a personal attack. We get to approach it with an open mind.

Chapter 24: Tips For A Less Stressful Day

So what about those small, daily stressful events that hinder us on a regular basis and cause us to feel down? Well, I've compiled a list of tips and that I'd like you to implement into your daily routine. A lot of these tricks have been shown to help with stress and anxiety. Depending on the person, some may work whilst others may not. Since everybody is different, there is no one solution to everyday stress. Some of these ideas can seem a little strange upon first hearing about them, but they work for a vast majority of people. So, keep an open mind and try them out. See which work for you and which don't.

I will say, don't try doing everything all at once though. Too much at one time can overhaul your life overnight. Focus on small changes, once a day, or once a week. Hopefully over time these small changes should add up and you'll find yourself in a better place.

Get familiar with your stress triggers

Recognize when you're having an anxiety attack, panic attack, or feeling stressed. A lot of people don't see the symptoms because they're not looking out for them. Just like an allergic reaction, you don't know what's causing it until something makes you pay attention. Notice the signs, which may include shallow breath, feeling lightheaded or nauseated, getting a headache, muscle tension, sweating, losing focus, feeling flushed, or unable to keep still. What was happening at the time to make you feel this way? What triggered the reaction? Make a list so that in the future, you can be better prepared to cope when these kind of situations come up again and deal with them. Just recognizing when you are feeling stressed can help you cope. The earlier you acknowledge it, the better you can control your feelings and actions in advance.

Understand when you are overreacting

Realize when you're overreacting. If you're prone to stressing and worrying too much then you know you've done this many times in the past. As often as you can, get a reality check so you know when you're overreacting. The fastest way to check yourself is ask a few other people: "am i overreacting?" If you can, stand back and look at a situation objectively. Is the situation really that bad? Is it a life or death situation? What is really the worst possible outcome? Learn to get perspective.

Find some quiet time

Once you notice you are feeling stressed, find a way to take a mini break from the stressful environment, situation, or person. Move away from the group, find privacy on a balcony, rest room, or go outside.

Breathe

Learn to control your breathing. This is the first exercise taught to students of meditation. Remember that stressed people tend to have shallow breaths, which makes the body lose oxygen very quickly, which may in turn lead to a full-blown panic attack. Take deep, slow breaths, focusing on the exhale, which will add oxygen to your blood. This increased oxygen has a relaxing effect on the body and is by far, the quickest, natural way to make us feel calm!

Lay down

If you can, lay down. Even if it's just laying on the floor. This position calms the heart, and keeps you still.

Get a regular massage

Some people respond very well to positive touch. A massage forces the body to relax, which can make the mind relax too. But if a massage does not work for you, and you only feel sore afterwards, don't worry about it.

All work and no play makes Jack a dull boy

Find a hobby you really enjoy. The mind needs to decompress regularly, and pursuing an activity you really get a kick out of might just be the perfect solution for you. Most of us just tend to watch TV, play computer games or surf the net when we need some down-time. But actually finding an activity that stimulates both your mind and body, has an overwhelmingly positive effect on your mental health. Spend some time exploring different activities until you find something that you can really get into.

Be creative

As human beings, our natural environment should be in a state of creativity. Depriving ourselves of this leaves us feeling flat and under-stimulated. Try to do something creative everyday or every week. This especially applies to creative people stuck in uncreative jobs. Find an outlet for your creativity. It doesn't have to be big. Maybe you could start a blog on a topic that interests you or start a Youtube channel documenting some interesting skills you might have. Maybe you could write a poem in the evening, or take up photography, programming, painting - the list is endless.

Make time for you

Make regular alone time. Especially effective for introverts with demanding social jobs or demanding households. Schedule time for yourself to relax alone and reflect events of the day.

Make time for others

On the flip side, you also have to make regular time for socializing. Effective for extroverts that wither on the vine when left alone too long. Seek out friends, even when you think you don't have the time.

Laugh

Find good humor. This could be a comedy show, funny movie, stand-up comic. Something that will make you laugh. Laughter actually decreases stress hormones, and helps tolerance to pain.

Variety is the spice of life

Go out and try something new. It could be a new restaurant, DIY project that caught your eye, discover new music, meet new people or read a new book. Those high in the Big Five openness trait get an actual emotional high in positive feelings from new experiences.

Exercise

Get fit. One of the major contributing factors of stress, anxiety and depression is simply down to a lack of exercise. Anatomically, we are designed to move. Sitting statically at a desk all day is not what we have been designed for. A lack of exercise may cause us to feel lethargic, run down and irritable whereas regular exercise tends to keep us feeling energized. Not only that, but regular exercise tends to increase endorphins (the body's feel-good hormone) and flushes out everything nasty, including toxins and stress hormones. Exercise is also the perfect way to blow off some steam. Think of your 30 minute run as detox for your mental health, not just something for your physical health. Exercise also increases your overall pain tolerance.

Eat a balanced diet

Make sure you eat regular and balanced meals, and drink enough water. You don't need to go on a complete health binge, just make sure you're not starving and that you're eating the right kind of food. It's important that you are getting enough vitamins and minerals into your daily diet. The best way to ensure this, is to make sure that you are consuming plenty of fruits and vegetables throughout the day. Science has proven that a lack of a balanced diet is a contributing factor to stress and mood. Likewise, consuming foods that may be considered "unhealthy" affect us negatively. In particular, foods high in sugar, fats and low in nutrition, actually spike our stress hormones. So, the food that you're eating could very well have a direct link to your levels of daily stress. A few simple adjustments then, might actually have a drastically beneficial effect. Something to consider. Nutritionally dense foods tend to make you feel good. Eating healthy will instantly elevate your mood and make you resistant to stress.

Sleep Well

Are you getting enough sleep? Sleep deprivation affects the brain more than you might think. It makes you more impulsive, more prone to poor decision making, irritable and fatigued. Unfortunately we live in a culture that considers 4-5 hours sleep a night the norm. This however, should not be considered normal at all. You should be aiming for (at least) 8 hours a night, on a regular basis. This may seem like a lot, however; you'd be surprised at how 8 hours of sleep affects overall health, mood and well-being. Try going to bed a few hours earlier than you usually would. If you find it hard sleeping, then try a few routines before turning in for the night. Switch off your electronics (cellphone, laptop, TV etc) early, get comfortable and read a book.

Skip the bad news.

Ever realize how the news always tends to report what's wrong with the world? Everyday it's all doom and gloom. The economy is crashing, wars, terrorism - the list is endless. Waking up and starting your morning with all this negativity sets you up the wrong way. Remove the news from your daily routine, as looking at this constantly will put you in a bad mood. You don't have to know what's happening all the time, especially if it does not directly affect you. If your life is already overwhelming, don't bother reading the papers or following news outlets.

Get a pet

Bring a furry friend into your life. Playing, stroking or talking to a pet can reduce stress. Many therapists (around three quarters) will recommend their patients adopt a pet. Pet therapy does work for many, but not all people. If you're not an animal lover, then its probably best to skip this one.

Get spiritual

A University Of Toronto study in 2009 was able to show that a spiritual practice, especially one taught in childhood, can bring order to your mind, and relieve excessive stress and worry. Good news then if you already have a spiritual practice - just get more in tune with your beliefs. And for those that aren't religious? Well, you can still be spiritual by practicing mindfulness, meditation or finding a philosophy that's in-line with your core beliefs. Just be wary of any any cults or extremist movements when going down this path.

Don't over-stimulate your brain

Avoid coffee, chocolates, red bull, pre-workout and other stimulants. If your nerves are already on edge, caffeine will only make them worse. It may be time to take these things out of your diet completely.

Nobody is perfect

Don't try to be a perfectionist. Seeking perfection can be stressful, and even paralyzing. Instead, aim for good enough. When starting something new, don't stress over failing to achieve perfection.

You want excellence sure, and that will come with time. Practice, and many mistakes that build up to improvements will eventually lead to achieving excellence in your work.

Things don't have to be so complicated

Simplify your life. Feeling overwhelmed can cause extreme stress. While some stress can be good motivation, too much stress will break you. So when you are feeling overwhelmed, don't hesitate to take a step back. If possible, take on less work responsibilities, simplify your schedule and to-do lists or just learn to say no. If you have a huge task that seems like a mountain to climb - then break it down into steps and work from there.

Lets say you have a large amount of dept which needs to be paid off. This can seem like an impossible task at first, unachievable. If you break it down however, the task seems less complicated than it actually needs to be. Get out a pen and piece of paper and brainstorm all the steps you should take to reach your goal.

Step 1 might be to cut up your credit cards. Step 2 could be work out a monthly budget. Step 3 could be to give up some unnecessary spending (like the daily Starbucks). Step 4 could be setting up a separate savings account which has a limited withdrawal amount. Step 5 could be making a list of methods for extra income.

Taking the time to sit down and plan out all the steps required to accomplish a large task, allows the brain to see the end goal and visually plans out a road map to our destination. This can really do wonders for stress / anxiety.

Declutter

Go minimal, reduce the clutter in your living space. This can be especially difficult if you are a hoarder or collector. Your physical space reflects your inner state of mind. If your space is disorganized, overflowing with too much going on, so is your mind. It's a huge task to declutter and keep tidy, but worth the effort in keeping a peaceful mind.

Borrow someone's ear

Find the right person to listen to you. Not everybody is worth sharing your problems with of course, but if you have somebody to talk to, it can help a lot. Talking to someone who is understanding and compassionate can relieve a lot of negative emotions. Talking to somebody logical and objective, can help organize your thoughts and even find solutions you would not think of yourself. Don't talk to somebody negative or critical as they may make you feel worse. If you have a trusted friend or family member though, sharing your feelings can be extremely beneficial.

Let off some some steam

Take a hot bath or shower. You could also try a sauna session, an ice bath, or hot and cold therapy where you alternate between hot and cold water. The sudden change in temperature makes the muscles relax, easing pain and tension that can be caused by stress. The effect is instant, and in some cases, can be more effective than taking medication.

Running water

Seek water, some people find the sound of flowing water very soothing. Buy a mini desk fountain, download a track of the sound of crashing waves, go for a swim, walk by a lake or stream. The sound of water can help people feel calm and more creative. Interestingly, studies have shown that people who live by the ocean have lower stress levels than those who don't. Go figure!

Ambience

Turn to music. People have different tastes in music, but for stress relief, try ambient music, which has been shown to reduce stress for up to 60% in those who listen to it. There's a reason ambient music is used in spas and yoga classes.

Get flexible

Try a yoga class. There are several kinds of yoga, and different kinds of teachers. Find a teacher and environment that suits you. Yoga reconnects the body and mind, and helps you become acutely aware of your breathing and the movement of your muscles during class. This training helps you take control over your body, mind and over time can help you to have more control over your stress levels.

Seek out nature

Spend 20 minutes a day outdoors, especially when it's a good day. Exposure to the sun and greenery affects your mood. This is an inherited response from our human ancestors who spent all day outside. If you've ever experience long winter months, you'll understand how important natural sunlight is to your mood.

Being in nature, with green all around is just as important as sunlight. You can actually induce relaxation by just looking at the color green, even if it's on your desktop screen or the color of your walls. However, this is not a substitution for just going outside, walking around a garden or park.

Pierce the problem

Try acupuncture. This method can be intimidating if you've never tried it before. But don't worry, it's perfectly safe! There are studies that show acupuncture to be effective for treating pain relief. It can also be used to make you release certain hormones to relax. There are no serious side effects to using acupuncture, aside from small pin prick marks on the skin. It could be worth your time, especially if you want to avoid strong side effects from conventional medications.

CPSIA information can be obtained
at www.ICGtesting.com
Printed in the USA
BVHW041624300520
580482BV00011B/417

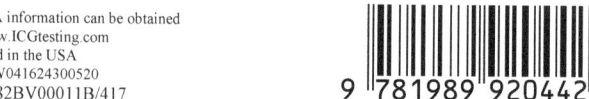